MILADY'S AESTHETICIAN SERIES

Common Drugs and Side Effects: A Handbook for the Aesthetician

MILADY'S AESTHETICIAN SERIES

Common Drugs and Side Effects: A Handbook for the Aesthetician

PAMELA HILL, R.N.

THOMSON
DELMAR LEARNING

Australia Canada Mexico Singapore Spain United Kingdom United States

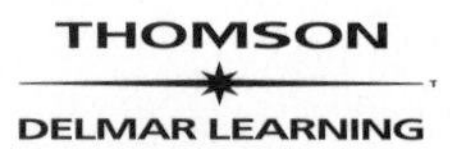

Milady's Aesthetician Series: Common Drugs and Side Effects—A Handbook for the Aesthetician

Pamela Hill

President, Milady:
Dawn Gerrain

Managing Editor:
Robert Serenka

Acquisitions Editor:
Martine Edwards

Product Manager:
Jennifer Anderson

Editorial Assistant:
Falon Ferraro

Director of Content and Media Production:
Wendy A. Troeger

Content Project Manager:
Nina Tucciarelli

Composition:
Pre-PressPMG

Director of Marketing:
Wendy Mapstone

Director Beauty Industry Relations
Sandra Bruce

Marketing Coordinator:
Nicole Riggi

Text Design:
Essence of Seven

Printed in United States
1 2 3 4 5 XXX 11 10 09 08 07

For more information contact Thomson Delmar Learning,
5 Maxwell Drive,
CLIFTON PARK, NY 12065-2919
at http://www.milady.com

Library of Congress Cataloging-in-Publication Data

Hill, Pamela, RN.
Common drugs and side effects : a handbook for the aesthetician/Pamela Hill.
p. ; cm. -- (Milady's aesthetician series)
Includes bibliographical references and index.
ISBN-13: 978-1-4018-8172-6
ISBN-10: 1-4018-8172-6
1. Drugs--Side effects--Handbooks, manuals, etc. 2. Dermatotoxicology--Handbooks, manuals, etc.
3. Pharmacology--Handbooks, manuals, etc. I. Title. II. Series: Hill, Pamela, RN. Milady's aestetician series.
[DNLM: 1. Drug Eruptions--Handbooks. 2. Pharmaceutical Preparations--adverse effects--Handbooks. 3. Skin--drug effects--Handbooks. 4. Skin Manifestations--Handbooks.
WR 165 H647c 2008]
RM302.5.H55 2008
615'.7042--dc22
2007002850

Contents

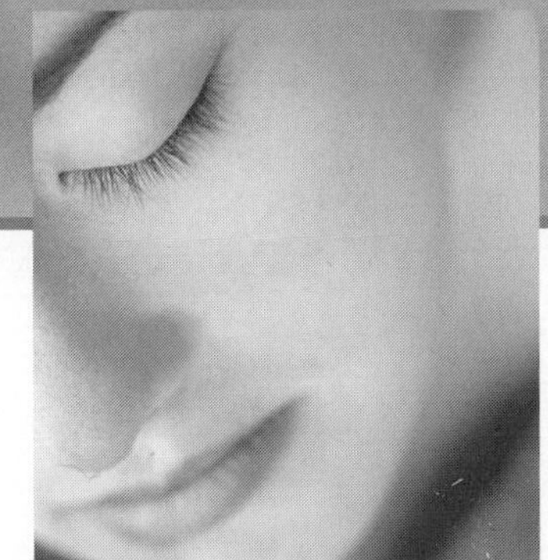

CHAPTER 3

CHAPTER 4

CHAPTER 5

CHAPTER 8

CHAPTER 9

CHAPTER 10

Preface

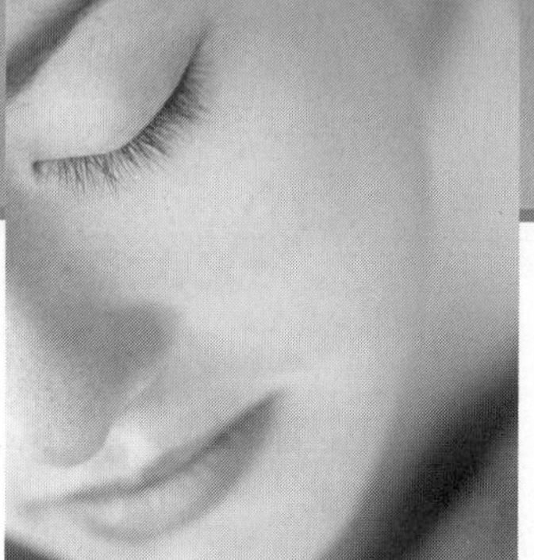

Almost daily a clinician will find herself looking at an intake sheet and wondering about the drugs a patient is taking. What are they for? Do they affect the skin? Will the products used for a treatment cause a reaction? Does the drug cause skin sensitivity? These questions and more should give a good clinician pause and send her to look up the drug. But that is easier said than done. Not all facilities have a PDR (physician's desk reference), and often the information contained in a book like the PDR is confusing and difficult to disseminate.

This book will help the aesthetician quickly reference the drug(s) that a patient is taking. Diseases and the drugs that improve life can easily have an effect on the skin. And while an aesthetician's job does not include medication management or disease management, it is important for him/her to understand a little bit about diseases and the drugs that improve the quality of a patient's life. The more the clinician knows about her clients the easier it is to manage their skin care.

This book does not provide in-depth information about drugs. The text is concise and directed to the aesthetician's needs. It is in an easy format for a clinician to use, with each drug listed by the generic name. Only the ***most common side effects*** have been listed; however, all of the ***possible skin effects*** have been included.

The book is organized by drug category with a cross-referenced glossary, making it easy to resource a drug by trade name or generic name. It should be noted that this book is NOT inclusive of all drugs available. Some drugs that are given only by intravenous routes or intramuscular routes may not have been included. Furthermore, drugs that are experimental or infrequently used may have been deleted.

For an aesthetician, regardless of the area of expertise, knowledge is power. Understanding the basics of a disease and the medications that are used to manage the problem will help the aesthetician to make the treatments in a spa safer. This book is designed for just that purpose—to lower the bar to entry, if you will—so that the aesthetician feels comfortable accessing information and improving the care for the client.

About the Author

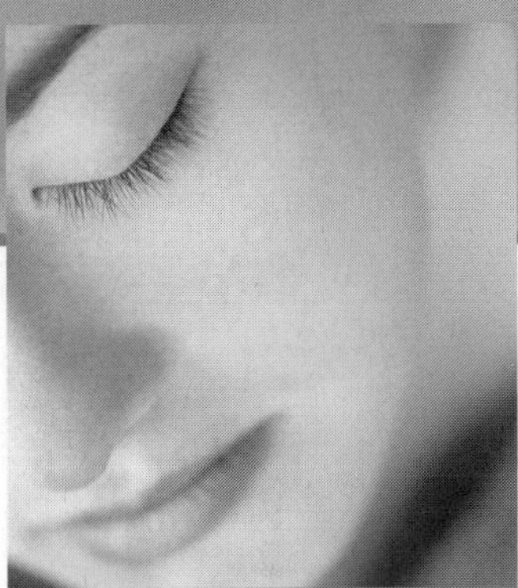

Pamela Hill received her nursing diploma from Presbyterian Hospital and Colorado Women's College, Denver, Colorado, and has practiced as a registered nurse for more than 20 years. Her background includes 15 years of operational and leadership experience in the medical spa, medical skin care, and educational sector. Ms. Hill has been instrumental in the growth and development of Facial Aesthetics, Inc. ("FAI"), a successful Colorado-based medical spa. An astute results-oriented leader with a proven track record of building and growing companies in the medical appearance sector, she has been actively involved in the evolution of the medical spa model as well as the research and development of the Pamela Hill Skin Care product line. Ms. Hill has been active with patient care, the development of policy and procedure, and clinician education. Passionate about the education of aestheticians in the medical spa setting, Ms. Hill began a relationship with Milady, an imprint of Delmar Learning, in 2003. This relationship launched Ms. Hill's authoring of the Aesthetician Series, a twelve book series dedicated to the education of medical aestheticians and the must-have information for on-the-job success. Currently six of the books are in print.

Ms Hill has appeared on national and regional radio talk shows, including "Here's to your Health," and has been quoted in the *Denver Post, Rocky Mountain News,* and *Beverly Hills' 213.*

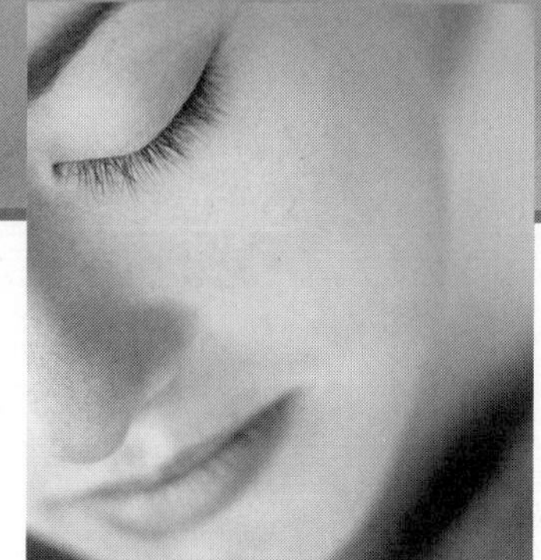

Acknowledgments

Writing a book is a collaborative effort. It involves not only the author, the editors, the production team, the marketing team, and the composition team but also the reviewers. The best books come together when the reviewers provide honest, constructive feedback that can be implemented into the manuscript to improve the book. In this particular case I was lucky to have a group of reviewers that helped me to improve the quality of this book. A special thank you goes to the reviewers who spent their precious leisure time reviewing this book.

As always a big thank you to my beacon of light: my husband, John.

Reviewers

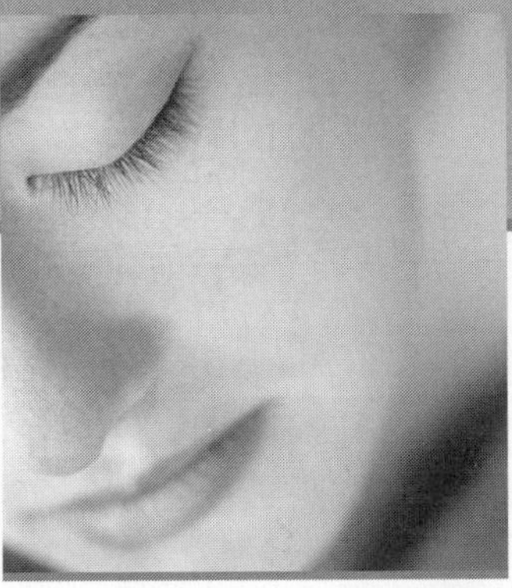

The author and publisher would like to thank the following individuals who have reviewed this text and offered invaluable feedback. This very important task, although time-consuming for each reviewer, is a critical component to the success of a book. We are grateful for your time and honest comments.

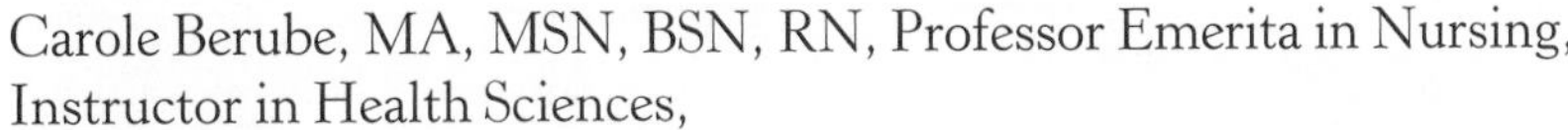

Carole Berube, MA, MSN, BSN, RN, Professor Emerita in Nursing, Instructor in Health Sciences,
Bristol Community College, Fall River, Massachusetts

Felicia Brown, LMBT,
Beyond Bodywork Solutions, Greensboro, North Carolina

Karen S. Columbus, MMA, MA,
Skin Dynamics Research

Stephanie Garthrite, CPhT,
Remington College, Cleveland, Ohio

Nancy Hemmings Owens, Instructor,
Daytona, Brevard and Mitchell Community College

James J. Mizner Jr., BS Pharmacy, RPh, MBA,
ACT College, Arlington, Virginia

Sandra Peoples,
Pickens Technical Center, Aurora, Colorado

Introduction

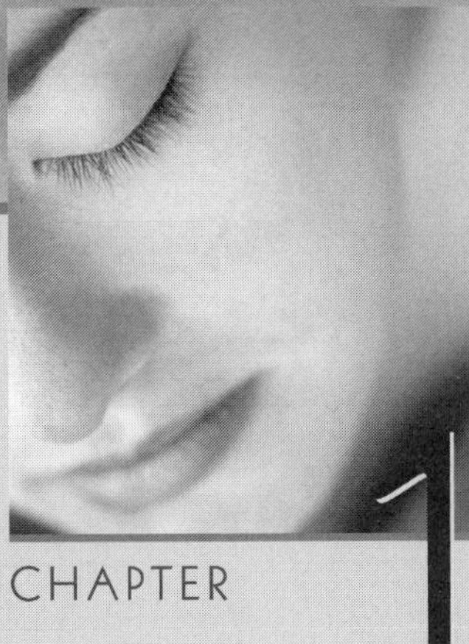

CHAPTER 1

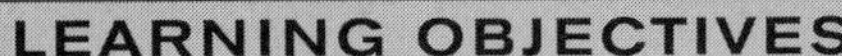

KEY TERMS

Food and Drug Administration (FDA)
Health History Sheet
Hyperpigmentation
Hypopigmentation
Over-the-counter (OTC)
Prescription

LEARNING OBJECTIVES

After completing this chapter, you should be able to:

1. Explain the FDA.
2. Define a prescription.
3. Discuss who can write a prescription.

An aesthetician's job does not include medication management or disease management; this is the territory of the physician. However, as aestheticians, we can be in situations where we need to understand the medication a client is taking. Sometimes, what we see on the surface of the skin is a function of the drugs a patient is taking. If we do not reference this drug, how will we know? Will our procedures make these side effects worse? Will the healing be impaired? Will the products we recommend for home care inflame the skin or open the skin to infection? These are questions we should ask ourselves when we see the patient intake sheet and find drugs listed that we do not recognize.

Given that the clinician is not in the position of prescribing medication, managing medications, or diagnosing disease, these topics are not covered; this book is intended as a quick reference. Each drug category is identified, followed by some of the more common drugs in that category. Also included are the trade name, side effects, and skin side effects. This allows the clinician an opportunity to become more educated about the medication category and its purpose and potential side effects.

INTRODUCTION

over-the-counter (OTC)
a medication that is available for consumption without a physician's prescription

prescription
a doctor's order for a medication to remedy an illness or the symptoms of an illness

hyperpigmentation
overproduction and overdeposits of melanin

hypopigmentation
lack of production of melanin from melanocytes

As early as 100 years ago, medicines, whether **over-the-counter** or **prescription,** did not exist as we know them today. In fact, antibiotics have only actively been used since World War II. But times are changing, and one of the major therapeutic modalities is by means of prescription medicines.

As an aesthetician, you will obviously not be able to write prescriptions. Only certain qualified medical personnel such as doctors, physician assistants, and nurse practitioners may prescribe drugs. But many of the prescribed drugs may have side effects and consequences that affect the outcomes of the treatments that you will be providing. For instance, the use of certain drugs may be contraindicated for a specific treatment or may be the source of **hyperpigmentation** or **hypopigmentation.**

To better serve your clients and your career, it is important to be actively involved in seeking out information from your clients. The best opportunity to do this is during the consultative process when you will be learning about your clients, their skin care goals, and, relevant to this text, their health histories.

The **Health History Sheet** asks for a detailed health status. This questionnaire probes into the past and current health of your patient. Included on this document are questions about allergies, current and past illnesses, smoking status, pregnancy status, daily medications, and past surgical events. The objective of the health history is to obtain a detailed "snap shot" of the client's health. This form should be set up in a check-box format. While the client may think that some of the health items are irrelevant, the questions may be important in delivering care, and all items should have a "yes" or "no" box checked. This document may also give you an idea of why the patient is seeking a particular treatment. This information is all vital and should be as accurate and complete as possible.

Once you have a complete list of the drugs that your patient is taking, you should take a moment and cross reference the medication skin effects with the skin complaints for which the patient requests care. If you suspect that his or her complaints are a result of the medications being used, you should discuss this with the client. Discontinuing a prescribed medication because of its effect on the skin (such as hyperpigmentation) is absolutely wrong. In fact, an aesthetician should never make this recommendation. You may, however, suggest that your client consult his or her physician to discuss the possibility of finding a medication that does not so adversely affect the skin.

Health History Sheet
document used by medical professionals to gather information on past and present health conditions, as well as likelihood for future conditions. This includes allergies, medical conditions, and prescription information

Food and Drug Administration (FDA)
regulatory agency of the federal government which oversees drugs currently on the market and approves drugs for consumption

FDA AND DRUGS

As part of the Department of Health and Human Services, **The Food and Drug Administration (FDA)** is tasked with making sure that drugs that reach the marketplace are safe for consumption. This is done by approving drugs through holding trials, regulating labeling, and monitoring drugs that are already on the market. The FDA requires this process for both prescription and nonprescription medications.

The FDA as we now know it was established in 1938, following the deaths of dozens of people who ingested an elixir that was heavily fortified with a poisonous agent. Public outcry led to the passage of the Federal Food, Drug, and Cosmetic Act. This law resulted in the formation of the FDA, creating a new drug application (NDA) and required clinical studies be performed on potential drug identities before they can be introduced into the marketplace. New drugs must undergo a four phase clinical trial process prior to release, involving thousands of people and often taking years to complete.

The FDA is subject to political and public scrutiny. Those who oppose the FDA argue that they prevent lifesaving medications from becoming available and often act in favor of political motives versus scientific ones, driving up overall health care costs. Those who support the FDA argue that its policies and procedures save many more lives than the drugs it does not approve. Whatever your opinion, suffice it to say that the FDA will not be eliminated anytime soon.

The procedures for gaining FDA approval are complex, but can be summed up by saying that provided that a new drug is safe for consumption, and it works as well as or better than similar products on the market, it will achieve FDA approval. A patent is issued to the manufacturer for each drug approved by the FDA. Those products approved before June 8, 1995, had a 17 year patent, while those approved after that date received a 20 year patent.[1]

During this period, only the originating manufacturer can produce the drug. This gives that manufacturer authority to establish prices and drive the demand. Following the expiration of the patent, other pharmaceutical companies can start making generic versions of the same product.

While the FDA approves new drugs, monitors old ones, and performs quality checks on the labeling and purity of food and drugs, it does not regulate cosmetics or herbal products.

The Approval of Prescription Drugs

The drug approval process is one that is long, complicated, expensive, and time-consuming. On average, it costs in excess of 500 million dollars to get a drug from conception to approval, and all of this money is spent without the guarantee of FDA approval. Only one out of every 5000 drugs that undergo pretrial evaluation will ever achieve FDA approval. Only five of these drugs will ever be tested on humans. The drug approval process in the United States is the strictest in the world.

Once researchers develop a compound that is suspected to have the desired effect, the pretrial testing begins. This is done in a laboratory, usually on animals, computer models, and tissue, but not on living human test subjects. This is a long process, usually taking as many as four years. This is because, before it is tested on healthy human beings, it needs to prove that it will not be of detriment to the human subjects and that it has proven effective at its intended goal. Once that is complete, a request is submitted to the FDA to begin testing on human subjects, which is called Investigational New Drug Testing.

Once pretrial testing has proven to be worthwhile, it begins an arduous multiphased trial process. There are three phases of testing with specific objectives in each test phase. Among the test objectives are efficacy, dosage, side effects, as well as long term positive and negative

[1]http://www.fda.gov

results. Once all three phases of testing are complete and the results are compiled, the drug is submitted for FDA approval. If the drug is approved, a postapproval test phase will begin.

PRESCRIPTION DRUGS

Once approved by the FDA these drugs are then available for physicians to prescribe to their patients. A prescription requires the supervision of a physician, while an OTC (over-the-counter) medication does not. A prescription requires a physician's "order," which includes the name, strength, and quantity of the medication as well as appropriate directions for use. If the medication is safe to use without a physician's supervision, it is classified as a nonprescription or OTC product and can be purchased at a local drug store or supermarket.

Definition of a Prescription

A prescription is defined as a physician's order for and recommended administration of a particular drug. Originally, ancient prescriptions were composed of a detailed list of ingredients that when combined formed a complex preparation. These recipes were often written in codes to protect the secrets of their purposes. Today, a universal language and process is used to write prescriptions. The process has a common format: patient information, symbol Rx (which comes from the Latin) meaning "recipe," Signatura, which is the body of the prescription and means instructions to the patient, and finally the signature of the prescribing physician. In modern America, prescription writing privileges for controlled

for ______________________ *date* ______________

R_x

______________________ *M.D.* ○ *Label* *Refill* *Times*

Confirm DEA & License # for telephone prescriptions requests.

Figure 1-1 Illustration of a prescription blank

substances are regulated by the Drug Enforcement Agency. This process is granted only to specific individuals in the medical, veterinary, and dental world. Those who are given this privilege are physicians, dentists, physician's assistants, and nurse practitioners. In some states optometrists have limited prescription authority to write prescriptions for eyeglasses. In all states prescriptions include the DEA number (for controlled substances), and in some states a prescriber's license number is required. Forgery of prescriptions is taken very seriously.

Common Prescription Drugs

The aesthetician should be aware of the common prescription drug categories that might be presented by a client. These oral drugs typically treat the diseases we read about each day such as diabetes, heart disease, depression, and bacterial and viral infections. Those over-the-counter drugs that the aesthetician might see on the intake form include pain medications or cold and flu medications and allergy medications.

Topical prescription products may be more common to the aesthetician and include categories such as antiaging, antibiotic, antiviral, and anti-inflammatory drugs.

OVER-THE-COUNTER DRUGS

Over-the-counter medications are those that treat common conditions, yet they do not require a prescription from a physician. These products

Table 1-1 Common Oral Prescription Drugs

Category of Drug	Common Drug Names	Common Reasons for the Prescription
Antidepressants	Prozac, Zoloft	Depression
Antivirals	Zovirax, Valtrex	Herpes simplex (cold sores)
Antibiotics	Tetracycline	Acne or infections
Antifungals	Lamisil	Fungal infections
Diuretics	Hydrochlorothiazide	Hypertension
Hormones	Estrogen	Menopause
Hypoglycemic agents	Actos, Glucophage	Diabetes

Table 1-2 Common Topical Prescription Drugs

Category of Drug	Common Drug Names	Common Reasons for the Prescription
Antiaging	Renova	Lines and wrinkles
Antibiotics	Cleocin T	Acne
Antivirals	Denavir	Cold sores
Anti-inflammatory	Aclovate	Irritation from peel or treatment

Table 1-3 Common Over-the-Counter Drugs

Category of Drug	Common Use	Common Products
Antiaging Medications	Accelerated epidermal turnover	Glycolic acid
Pain Medications	Reduce minor pain	Motrin
Antidiarrheal Medications	Treat minor diarrhea	Imodium AD

are still regulated by the FDA, but are proven safe enough for public consumption without the oversight required by a prescription.

The safety of the over-the-counter product is provided by the labeling. As part of its ongoing mission to protect the health of Americans with regard to drugs, the FDA requires that all over-the-counter medications list the same required information, in the same order, so that it is easier to see ingredients of the product, directions for use, and other pertinent information. Common over-the-counter drugs that the aesthetician might find on the intake form of a potential client include antiaging medications, pain medications, and antidiarrheal medications

DRUG CATEGORIES

Drug categories are definitions for a group of drugs. The category is basically an umbrella for the group of drugs that provide the same or a similar effect. According to the FDA, there are over 35 drug categories. Among those categories that we will be examining are the following: analgesics, antianxiety drugs, antiarrhythmics, antibiotics, anticonvulsants,

Table 1-4 Drug Categories

Drug Category	Expected Result	Example of a Drug in this Category
Analgesics (narcotic and non-narcotic)	Relieve pain	Narcotic: Morphine Non-Narcotic: Aspirin
Antacids	Relieve indigestion	TUMS
Antianxiety	Relieve anxiety	Xanax
Antiarrhythmics	Control the heartbeat	Tikosyn, Ethmozine
Antibiotics	Treat infections	Ceclor
Anticoagulants	Prevent blood clotting	Coumadin
Anticonvulsants	Prevent seizures	Tegretol, Dilantin
Antidepressants	Lift mood	Wellbutrin
Antidiarrheals	Relieve diarrhea	Lomotil
Antiemetics	Treat nausea and vomiting	Zofran
Antifungals	Treat fungal infections	Lamisil
Antihistamines	Counteract effects of histamine	Benadryl
Antihypertensives	Lower blood pressure	Zestril
Anti-inflammatories	Reduce inflammation	Motrin, Naprosyn
Antineoplastics	Treat cancer	Hexalen
Antipsychotics	Treat psychotic disorders	Thorazine
Antipyretics	Reduce fever	Acetaminophen
Beta-Blockers	Reduce the oxygen needs of heart by reducing heart rate	Lopressor
Bronchodilators	Open the bronchial tubes	Proventil
Corticosteroids	Anti-inflammatories for arthritis or asthma	Medrol Dose Pak
Cough Suppressants	Reduce cough	HOLD Lozenges
Cytotoxics	Kill cells; used to treat cancer	Tamoxifen

Table 1-4 Drug Categories

Drug Category	Expected Result	Example of a Drug in this Category
Decongestants	Reduce membrane swelling	Sudafed
Diuretics	Increase urine	Lasix
Expectorants	Promote coughing	Mucinex
Hormones	Provide hormone replacement therapy	Estrogen, Progesterone
Hypoglycemics	Reduce blood glucose	Glucophage
Immunosuppressives	Treat autoimmune diseases	Azathioprine
Laxatives	Increase bowel movements	Metamucil
Muscles Relaxants	Relieve muscles spasms	Flexeril
Sleep Drugs	Work as sedatives	Ambien
Thrombolytics	Help to dissolve clots	Heparin
Vitamins	Provide chemicals essential for good health	Vitamin C, A

antidepressants, antifungals, antihistamines, antihypertensives, anti-inflammatories, antineoplastics, antipsychotics, bronchodilators, corticosteroids, diuretics, hormones, hypoglycemics, and muscle relaxants. In each category there are many drugs that provide the same treatment. Multiple drugs have been developed in each category to address the potential allergies of clients as well as the possible efficacy of one drug over another.

Conclusion

The use of prescription drugs is familiar in our society. Whether treating an infection or managing a disease process, a patient taking prescription drugs will be a familiar situation for the practicing aesthetician. The aesthetician's role is to understand what drugs are being used and for what reason. Furthermore, it is important for the aesthetician to understand the effect certain drugs have on the skin and consequently on the treatments a client might be receiving. Keeping alert and watching for possible skin effects is a role the clinician must accept and take responsibility for.

REFERENCES

1. http://www.nlm.nih.gov
2. http://www.rxlist.com
3. http://www.drugs.com
4. Michalun, N. (2001). *Milady's Skin Care and Cosmetic Ingredients Dictionary.* Clifton Park: Thomson Delmar Learning.
5. Spratto, G.R., and Woods, A.L. (2005). *2005 PDR Nurse's Drug Handbook.* Clifton Park: Thomson Delmar Learning.
6. http://www.fda.gov

Anti-Parkinson and Anti-Alzheimer's Drugs

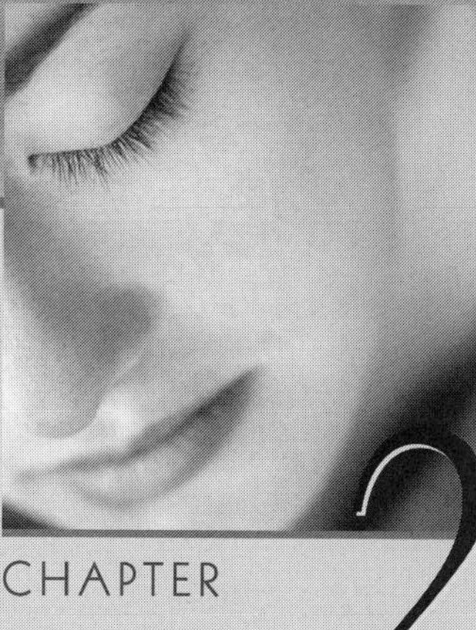

CHAPTER 2

KEY TERMS

Anticholinergics
Acetylcholinesterase
Alzheimer's Disease
Catechol-0-Methyltransferase Inhibitors
Ecchymoses
Parkinson's Disease
Photosensitivity

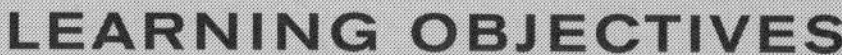

LEARNING OBJECTIVES

After completing this chapter, you should be able to:

1. Define Alzheimer's disease and discuss the progression of the disease.
2. Define Parkinson's disease and discuss the progression of the disease.
3. Discuss pharmaceutical options for Alzheimer's and Parkinson's diseases.

INTRODUCTION

Alzheimer's disease
chronic, progressive neurological condition characterized by early onset of dementia

Parkinson's disease
nervous system condition characterized by progressive tremors, muscular weakness, and rigidity

Alzheimer's disease and **Parkinson's disease** are degenerative diseases that render those who suffer from the symptoms victim to "good days" and "bad days." Currently, about 4.5 million people suffer from Alzheimer's disease. In the next 45 years, that number is expected to reach as high as 16 million.[1] Parkinson's disease, while not as common, affects 1.5 million in the United States at the present.[2] With certain exceptions, both of these diseases usually affect individuals over the age of 65. For the aspiring aesthetician, this means that at some point in your career, there is going to be a time when a client of yours will present with at least one of these conditions. For this reason, it is important to take special care to make certain that your clients' Health History Sheets are complete and accurate. The medications that these patients are on may have side effects that are important to bear in mind during an aesthetic treatment.

DRUGS USED FOR ALZHEIMER'S DISEASE AND DEMENTIA

As many as 4 million older Americans suffer from a form of dementia. Usually the effects of dementia begin to occur after the age of 60, and the risk increases greatly as the years pass. While it is extremely common in aging populations, most medical professionals agree that it is not a normal part of the aging process. Dementia is a brain disorder that seriously affects a person's ability to carry out daily activities. The most common form of dementia is Alzheimer's disease (AD), which initially involves the parts of the brain that control thought, memory, and language. While researchers are coming close to understanding the physiologic apparatuses that cause the condition, they are still far from finding a cure.

AD is named after Dr. Alois Alzheimer, a German doctor. In 1906, Dr. Alzheimer noticed changes in the brain tissue of a woman who had died of an unusual mental illness. He found abnormalities (now called amyloid plaques) and tangled bundles of fibers (now called neurofibrillary tangles) of brain tissue. Today, these plaques and tangles in the brain are considered signs of AD. These plaques, tangled fibers, and nerve cells die in areas of the brain that are vital to memory and other mental abilities, and connections between nerve cells are disrupted.

It is important to remember that an aesthetician has no authority to make any recommendations with regard to medications or dosages that a client uses. Always refer clients to their physicians if they cannot tolerate their medications.

[1]http://www.alzheimersinfo.org
[2]http://www.parkinsons.org

The medications used for AD increase the amount of acetylcholine in the central nervous system. Doing so helps to improve the patient's ability to reason, to use judgment, and to retain memory. While the cure has yet to be discovered, these medications serve to prolong the quality of life and memory of the patients who are afflicted with this condition.

Anti-Alzheimer's Drugs

donepezil Inhibits **acetylcholinesterase**, which may improve the dementia associated with AD, but will not alter the course of the disease

Side Effects: headache, diarrhea, nausea, vomiting, depression, dizziness, drowsiness
Trade Names: Aricept, Aricept ODT
Skin Effects: **ecchymoses**

acetylcholinesterase
enzyme that inhibits the activity of acetylcholine

ecchymoses
bruising

galantamine Enhances cholinergic function

Side Effects: fatigue, headache, fainting, slow heart rate, changes in eating patterns, nausea, vomiting, diarrhea, dyspepsia, weight loss, tremor
Trade Names: Razadyne, Razadyne ER
Skin Effects: none noted

memantine Prevents the binding of glutamate to a neurotransmitter

Side Effects: dizziness, fatigue, headache, changes in urination, changes in blood pressure, anemia
Trade Names: Namenda
Skin Effects: rash

rivastigmine Enhances the cholinergic function

Side Effects: weakness, anorexia, nausea, vomiting, tremor, dizziness, drowsiness, headache, gas, fever, upset stomach, weight loss
Trade Names: Exelon
Skin Effects: none noted

tacrine Increases acetylcholine

Side Effects: dizziness, headache, slow heart beat, anorexia, diarrhea, upset stomach, nausea, vomiting, GI bleeding (needs physician attention)
Trade Names: Cognex
Skin Effects: none noted

DRUGS USED TO TREAT PARKINSON'S DISEASE

Our brains are the complex powerhouses of our bodies. But in certain conditions particular brain cells can die, causing significant ramifications. In one such disease, Parkinson's disease, the brain cells that produce the important component known as dopamine no longer function. The chemical dopamine ensures that our movements flow evenly and with precision. Without dopamine, movements are jerky, movement is slow, and balance is affected. Parkinson's disease shows no favoritism—it affects men and women and all ethnicities. The treatment of Parkinson's is purely pharmaceutical; there is not a cure. The medications that are available simply mimic the production of dopamine, while others improve the rigidity and tremor associated with the disease.

Anti-Parkinson's Drugs

anticholinergics
drug class that acts to limit spasms and cramping, particularly of the digestive and urinary tracts

Catechol-0-Methyltransferase inhibitors
an agent that breaks down levodopa, allowing greater availability in the central nervous system

photosensitivity
condition characterized by increased sensitivity to light and the effects of light, particularly sunlight, on the skin

Anticholinergics and **Catechol-0-Methyltransferase** are the two main drug categories that are used in the treatment of Parkinson's disease. Anticholinergics allow more controlled muscle movements by relaxing the muscles and reducing stiffness, while Catechol-0-Methyltransferase inhibitors break down levodopa, allowing greater availability in the central nervous system.

Anticholinergics

benztropine Reduces muscle tremors by restoring the natural balance of neurotransmitters in the central nervous system

Side Effects: blurred vision, dry eyes, dry mouth, constipation, decreased sweating, changes in urination, fatigue, nausea, dizziness, fast heartbeat, headache, loss of memory, muscle cramps, anxiety, unusual excitement
Trade Names: Apo-Benztropine, Cogentin
Skin Effects: **photosensitivity**, skin rash

biperiden Reduces muscle tremors by restoring the natural balance of neurotransmitters in the central nervous system

Side Effects: blurred vision, dry eyes, dry mouth, constipation, decreased sweating, changes in urination, fatigue, nausea, dizziness, fast heartbeat, headache, loss of memory, muscle cramps, anxiety, unusual excitement
Trade Names: Akineton
Skin Effects: photosensitivity, skin rash

Catechol-0-Methyltransferase Inhibitors

entacapone Used in conjunction with levodopa and operates to optimize its usage by the body

Side Effects: liver damage, sleep disturbances, excessive dreaming, diarrhea, dizziness, vomiting, increased sweating, hallucinations, confusion, irregular heartbeat
Trade Names: Comtan
Skin Effects: sweating, bleeding in the dermal layer, skin tumors, alopecia

orphenadrine Skeletal muscle relaxant used for the treatment of tremors and stiffness

Side Effects: dryness of mouth, difficult or decreased urination, eye pain, fainting, fast or pounding heartbeat, abdominal pain, blurred vision, confusion, constipation, dizziness, drowsiness, excitement, irritability, nervousness, restlessness, headache, muscle weakness, nausea, trembling, enlarged pupils, hallucinations, breathing troubles, fatigue
Trade Names: Antiflex, Banflex, Flexoject, Flexon, Mio-Rel, Myolin, Myotrol, Norflex, Orfro, Orphenate
Skin Effects: skin rash, hives, itching, redness, sores, ulcers or white spots on lips or in mouth, swollen and/or painful glands, unusual bruising or bleeding

Adjunct Drugs Used to Treat Parkinson's Disease

Dopamine Agonists See Chapter 7

Monoamine Oxidase Type B Inhibitors See Chapter 7

dopamine agonists
any agent that increases dopamine activity

Conclusion

Many of the diseases associated with aging are inevitable, and, while troubling for the individuals afflicted, many of the drugs now on the market can prolong and improve life. Because some of the conditions are incurable and progressive, treatments for these conditions are complex and constantly evolving. Researchers and pharmaceutical companies invest billions of dollars each year with the hopes of finding drugs that will make conditions like Alzheimer's curable. Until then, treatments are available that will ease the suffering accompanied with these conditions.

It is important for the aesthetician to know that the medications used to treat these conditions are as varied as the conditions themselves. Along with the medications are a host of side effects and skin effects that could have repercussions for the treatments that you want to perform or the skin complaints of your clients.

It is vital to your outcomes that you attain a complete health history from your clients during the consultation process. This includes gathering a complete list of medications that correspond to the disorder. Cross-referencing these medications with their skin effects will help you to achieve an optimal outcome with regards to the services that you provide for the client.

REFERENCES

1. http://www.nlm.nih.gov
2. http://www.rxlist.com
3. http://www.drugs.com
4. Deglin, J.H., and Vallerand, A.H. (2007). *Davis's Drug Guide for Nurses.* Philadelphia, PA: F.A. Davis.
5. Michalun, N. (2001). *Milady's Skin Care and Cosmetic Ingredients Dictionary.* Clifton Park: Thomson Delmar Learning.
6. Spratto, G.R., and Woods, A.L. (2005). *2005 PDR Nurse's Drug Handbook.* Clifton Park: Thomson Delmar Learning.
7. http://www.fda.gov

Drugs that Affect the Blood

Lipid Lowering Agents, Thrombolytics, Anticoagulants, and Antiplatelets

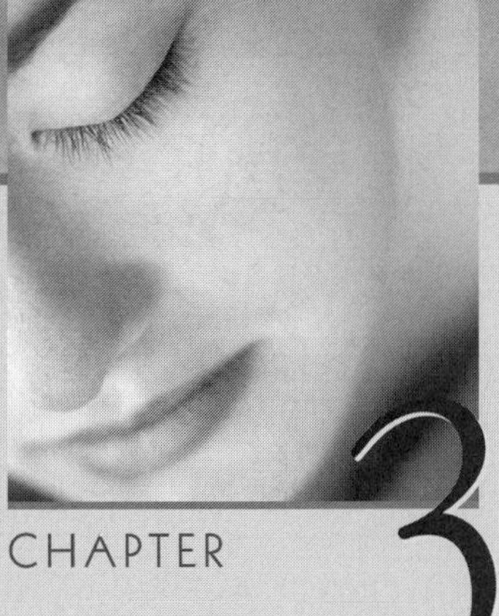

CHAPTER 3

KEY TERMS

Anaphylaxis
Cholecystitis
Cholelithiasis
Claudication
Hypercholesterolemia
Ischemic
Pancreatitis
Phlebitis
Primary Hypercholesterolemia
Prosthetic
Thrombocytopenia

LEARNING OBJECTIVES

After completing this chapter, you should be able to:

1. Describe platelets and their function.
2. Describe how lipids can cause heart attacks.

INTRODUCTION

The blood is one of the body's most interesting tissues. Yes, the blood is considered a tissue! While it appears thick and gooey to the naked eye, under the microscope, one can see the actual liquid and solid components. Depending on the amount of oxygen and carbon dioxide in the blood, the color will vary. The main constituents of blood are water, salts, plasma, and the substances transported by the blood. The cells that make up the blood include erythrocytes, leukocytes (5 types), and platelets. In this chapter we focus on two of the blood components: the platelets, which are involved in clotting, and fatty acids, one of the substances carried by the blood.

Blood Constituent
Water
Salts
Plasma
Substances transported by the blood

Blood Cells
Erythrocytes (red blood cells)
Leukocytes (white blood cells 5 types)
Platelets

LIPID LOWERING AGENTS

Cholesterol is normally found in the body in the cells of the nerves, muscles, skin, liver, intestines, and heart. There are three types of cholesterol found in the body: HDL, LDL, and VLDL. If the body has too much LDL cholesterol, the arteries become clogged. Cholesterol is especially attracted to the coronary arteries or those arteries that supply the heart its blood. High cholesterol increases the chances of heart disease. Consequently, elevated blood cholesterol may contribute to heart attacks. Therefore, a lot of attention has been given to the research and development of drug that lower lipids.

Bile Acid Sequestrants

Bile acid sequestrants are medications that deal primarily with **primary hypercholesterolemia**. They also manage excess bile acids. The mechanism of action is to bind the bile in the GI tract, in doing so the bile becomes unusable and is excreted. Bile acid sequestrants affect the low-density lipoproteins or LDL.

primary hypercholesterolemia the first in a series of events in which the affected individual presents with high cholesterol

cholestyramine

Side Effects: abdominal discomfort, constipation, nausea
Trade Names: LoCHOLEST, LoCHOLEST Light, Prevalite, Questran, Questran Light
Skin Effects: irritation and rashes

colesevelam

Side Effects: constipation and dyspepsia
Trade Names: Welchol
Skin Effects: none noted

colestipol

Side Effects: abdominal pain, constipation, nausea
Trade Names: Colestid
Skin Effects: irritation and rashes

HMG-COA Reductase Inhibitors

These drugs are commonly referred to as the "statins." This category includes one of the most familiar drugs used to treat high cholesterol, Lipitor. This medication (as others) should be used in conjunction with diet and exercise to lower the blood cholesterol. This medication interferes with an enzyme used to manufacture cholesterol.

atorvastatin

Side Effects: abdominal cramps, constipation, diarrhea, gas, heartburn
Trade Names: Lipitor
Skin Effects: rashes

fluvastatin

Side Effects: abdominal cramps, constipation, diarrhea, gas, heartburn

Trade Names: Lescol, Lescol XL
Skin Effects: rashes

lovastatin

Side Effects: abdominal cramps, constipation, diarrhea, gas, heartburn
Trade Names: Altocor, Altoprev, Mevacor
Skin Effects: rashes

pravastatin
Side Effects: abdominal cramps, constipation, diarrhea, gas, heartburn
Trade Names: Pravachol
Skin Effects: rashes

rosuvastatin
Side Effects: abdominal cramps, constipation, diarrhea, gas, heartburn
Trade Names: Crestor
Skin Effects: rashes

simvastatin
Side Effects: abdominal cramps, constipation, diarrhea, gas, heartburn
Trade Names: Zocor
Skin Effects: rashes

Other

This group of miscellaneous medications is used in combination with other lipid lowering agents to further reduce the cholesterol.

ezetimibe
Side Effects: **cholecystitis**, **cholelithiasis**, nausea, **pancreatitis**
Trade Names: Zetia
Skin Effects: rash

fenofibrate
Side Effects: fatigue, weakness
Trade Names: Antara, Lofibra, TriCor, Triglide
Skin Effects: rash

cholecystitis
inflammation of the gall bladder

cholelithiasis
formation of gallstones

pancreatitis
condition characterized by inflammation of the pancreas

gemfibrozil
Side Effects: abdominal pain, diarrhea, epigastric pain
Trade Names: Lopid
Skin Effects: alopecia, rashes, hives

niacin
Side Effects: upset stomach
Trade Names: Edur-Acin, Nia-Bid, Niac, Niacels, Niacor, Niaspan, Nicobid, Nico-400, Nicolar, Nicotinex, Nicotinic acid, Slo-Niacin Vitamin B
Skin Effects: itching, flushing of the face and neck, burning dry skin, hyperpigmentation, increased oiliness, rashes, tingling skin

niacinamide
Side Effects: upset stomach
Trade Names: Nicotinamide
Skin Effects: itching, flushing of the face and neck, burning dry skin, hyperpigmentation, increased oiliness, rashes, tingling skin

Omega 3 Acid Ethyl Esters
Side Effects: altered taste, gurgling in the stomach
Trade Names: Omacor
Skin Effects: rash

ANTICOAGULANTS

Anticoagulants are used to prevent the formation of clots. These medications are especially useful in the treatment of deep vein thrombosis, pulmonary embolism, and some heart problems. Anticoagulants will not dissolve clots that have already developed, but will help to prevent the clot from getting larger. This is why anticoagulants are used in combination with other medications such as antithrombotics to achieve the best result for the patient.

Antithrombotics

This medication is used to treat a variety of problems, including clots in the legs, secondary to **phlebitis**, and some heart problems. This medication works by prohibiting the clotting factors to proceed through their normal pathways.

phlebitis
inflammation of a vein

thrombocytopenia
abnormal decrease in blood platelet levels

anaphylaxis
serious hypersensitive allergic reaction characterized by respiratory distress, hypotension, edema, rash, and tachycardia. Immediate medical attention is necessary

heparin
Side Effects: anemia, **thrombocytopenia**
Trade Names: Hep-lock
Skin Effects: alopecia, rashes, hives

Coumarins

This medication is used to treat a variety of problems, including clots in the legs, secondary to phlebitis, and some heart problems. This medication works by interfering with the hepatic production of vitamin K. Coumarins are used to prevent blood clots.

warfarin
Side Effects: cramps, nausea, fever
Trade Names: Coumadin
Skin Effects: dermal necrosis

Thrombin Inhibitors

Thrombin inhibitors interfere with clotting activity by impeding the processes of thrombin.

argatroban
Side Effects: diarrhea, nausea, vomiting, fever
Trade Names: Argatroban
Skin Effects: none

bivalirudin
Side Effects: headache, hypotension, nausea, back pain, pain
Trade Names: Angiomax
Skin Effects: none

desirudin
Side Effects: nausea, anemia
Trade Names: Iprivask
Skin Effects: none

lepirudin
Side Effects: bleeding, **anaphylaxis**
Trade Names: Refludan
Skin Effects: none

Low Molecular Weight/Heparinoids

Low molecular weight/heparinoids are used for the treatment of **ischemic** stroke.

ischemic
temporary restriction in normal blood flow

dalteparin
Side Effects: anemia, thrombocytopenia
Trade Names: Fragmin
Skin Effects: ecchymoses, itching, rash, hives

enoxaparin
Side Effects: anemia, thrombocytopenia
Trade Names: Lovenox
Skin Effects: ecchymoses, itching, rash, hives

fondaparinux
Side Effects: anemia, thrombocytopenia
Trade Names: Arixtra
Skin Effects: ecchymoses, itching, rash, hives

tinzaparin
Side Effects: anemia, thrombocytopenia
Trade Names: Innohep
Skin Effects: ecchymoses, itching, rash, hives

ANTIPLATELETS

Platelets are blood cells that are involved in the clotting process. If an injury to the body occurs, platelets and other blood factors clump together, causing a clot to form. This process stops the bleeding. However, in some cases unwanted clots can occur. Antiplatelet drugs keep the platelets from becoming sticky preventing unwanted clots in the arteries or veins, including the vessels of the heart. These drugs are used to treat those individuals who are at risk of stroke or myocardial infarction. Antiplatelet drugs can also be used after certain types of surgery to prevent clots from forming. One of these surgeries might be cardiac surgery. Aspirin in low dosages is an antiplatelet drug.

Glycoprotein IIb/IIIa Inhibitors

Glycoprotein IIb/IIIa inhibitors are medications that are used to treat those individuals with certain types of heart conditions, specifically unstable angina or some heart attacks. Occasionally, at the discretion of the physician, these medications will be given in combination with other blood thinning agents such as an anticoagulant called heparin. As the aesthetician caring for a patient taking these medications, you need to know that the patient will bruise more easily. The treatment touch should be gentle to avoid any possible after bruising that the patient would consider disappointing to the treatment.

eptifibatide

Side Effects: Increased risk of side effects when the patient is taking heparin or aspirin in addition to this medication: hematomas, GI bleeding, hematuria, intracranial bleeding, hypotension
Trade Names: Integrilin
Skin Effects: bruising

tirofiban

Side Effects: headache
Trade Names: Aggrastat
Skin Effects: rash, hives

Platelet Adhesion Inhibitors

The platelet adhesion inhibitor is a medication that is typically used in combination with warfarin for the treatment of patients with **prosthetic** heart valves. This medicine will help to keep the prosthetic valve from accumulating small clots that might break away, causing serious problems.

prosthetic
replacement of a missing part with a man-made substitute

claudication
limping

dipyridamole

Side Effects: dizziness, headache, nausea
Trade Names: Persantine
Skin Effects: rash

Platelet Aggregation Inhibitors

These medications have several indications from the prevention of stroke to the treatment of **claudication**.

cilostazol

Side Effects: headache
Trade Names: Pletal
Skin Effects: none

clopidogrel

Side Effects: depression, dizziness, fatigue, headache, epistaxis, cough dyspnea, chest pain, edema, hypertension, abdominal pain, diarrhea, dyspepsia, gastritis, **hypercholesterolemia**, back pain, fever

Trade Names: Plavix

Skin Effects: rash, bruising, itching

hypercholesterolemia
condition characterized by abnormally high levels of cholesterol in the body

ticlopidine

Side Effects: diarrhea

Trade Names: Ticlid

Skin Effects: rashes, ecchymoses, hives, and itching

THROMBOLYTICS

Thrombolytics are used to degrade the fibrin found in clots. They are used in critical situations such as acute coronary thrombosis: clots in the vessels of the heart or clots in the lungs. These two examples are life-threatening situations. Thrombolytics are also used in the treatment of deep vein thrombosis. Thrombolytics can be used in conjunction with other medications that alter the clotting mechanisms; among those used in combination with thrombolytics might be aspirin, heparins, or warfarin.

alteplase

Side Effects: reperfusion arrhythmia

Trade Names: Activase, Cathflo Activase, tissue plasminogen activator (t-PA)

Skin Effects: ecchymoses, flushing, hives

anistreplase

Side Effects: reperfusion arrhythmia

Trade Names: anisoylated plasminogen-streptokinase activator complex (APSAC), Eminase

Skin Effects: ecchymoses, flushing, hives

reteplase

Side Effects: reperfusion arrhythmia

Trade Names: Retavase

Skin Effects: ecchymoses, flushing, hives

streptokinase

Side Effects: reperfusion arrhythmia

Trade Names: Kabikinase, Streptase

Skin Effects: ecchymoses, flushing, hives

tenecteplase

Side Effects: reperfusion arrhythmia
Trade Names: TNKase
Skin Effects: ecchymoses, flushing, hives

urokinase

Side Effects: reperfusion arrhythmia
Trade Names: Abbokinase
Skin Effects: ecchymoses, flushing, hives

Conclusion

Normally the blood provides our bodies with a healthy level of lipids and a normal process of clotting. But, as we now know, there are many circumstances in which these processes are interrupted. As an aesthetician caring for patients on these medications, you need to know that bruising is a possible side effect, and, consequently, it is important to be more gentle with the skin than you perhaps normally would be under different circumstances. Additionally, it is important for the aesthetician to encourage a healthy diet and exercise, not only for the blood lipid level, but also for the appearance of the skin.

REFERENCES

1. http://www.nlm.nih.gov
2. http://www.rxlist.com
3. http://www.drugs.com
4. Deglin, J.H., and Vallerand, A.H. (2007). *Davis's Drug Guide for Nurses*. Philadelphia, PA: F.A. Davis.
5. Michalun, N. (2001). *Milady's Skin Care and Cosmetic Ingredients Dictionary.* Clifton Park: Thomson Delmar Learning.
6. Spratto, G.R., and Woods, A.L. (2005). *2005 PDR Nurse's Drug Handbook*. Clifton Park: Thomson Delmar Learning.
7. http://www.fda.gov

Drugs that Affect the Heart
Antianginals and Antiarrythmics

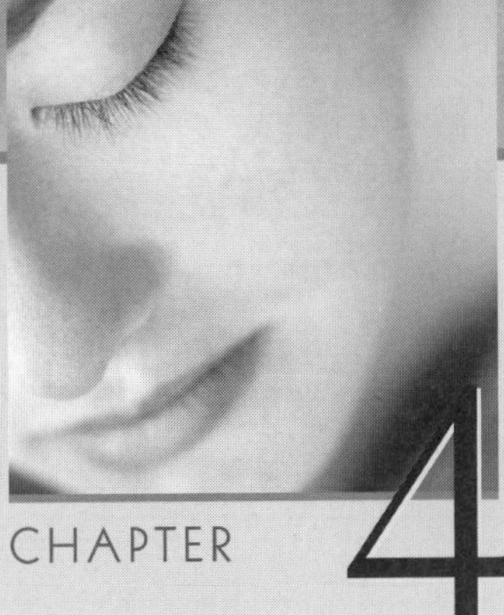

CHAPTER 4

KEY TERMS

Acute Coronary Syndrome
Angina
Antianginals
Ataxia
Atrial Flutter
AV Conduction
Erythema Multiforme
Hypertension
Hypertrichosis
Lethargy
Myocardial Ischemia
Normal Sinus Rhythm
Nystagmus
Parenterally
Peripheral Edema
Pruritus
Sublingually
Urticaria
Ventricular Arrhythmia
Ventricular Tachycardia

LEARNING OBJECTIVES

After completing this chapter, you should be able to:

1. Identify the most common heart diseases.
2. Discuss the different medications used to treat common heart diseases.

INTRODUCTION

Our bodies begin to deteriorate much sooner than many of us would like. Our hearts, for example, as steady and reliable as they are, are prone to wear and tear, especially if proper diet and exercise have not been part of our daily routine, not to mention the effects of stress associated with everyday life. Heart problems could include rhythm disruptions (arrthymias), **hypertension**, and, the deadliest of all, **acute coronary syndrome**. Acute coronary syndrome is an umbrella term that is used to describe those problems associated with blood flow to the heart. Just as other muscles need blood flow directed specifically to the muscle, so does the heart. When that blood flow is blocked or compromised in any way, acute coronary syndrome or **myocardial ischemia** occurs. Acute coronary syndrome accounts for one-third of all deaths among Americans, making it the nation's leading killer.

hypertension
high blood pressure

acute coronary syndrome (ACS)
general term used for any condition that causes chest pain resulting from limited blood flow to the heart

myocardial ischemia
temporary restriction in normal blood flow to the heart and cardiac muscles

angina
chest pain resulting from lack of oxygen supplied to the heart

Strokes are also a cardiovascular disease but are inclusive of the arteries in the brain rather than the heart. According to the National Stroke Association, strokes are the third largest killer and the number one disabler of Americans. After age 55, the rate of strokes doubles with each 10 years of age. Risk factors include ethnic considerations (African Americans have a greater incidence), age, smoking, and high blood pressure. And while men are more commonly affected than women, it is still important for women to be aware of the symptoms of stroke and act immediately.

ANGINA

Angina is the medical term for chest pain. It is a condition that should be taken very seriously. Angina is a symptom of myocardial ischemia or lack of blood flow to the heart. It is often mistaken for a heart attack. While not as deadly, it could be considered a symptom of heart disease. It may feel like pressure or a squeezing pain in the chest. The pain may also occur in the shoulders, arms, neck, jaw, or back. It could also feel like indigestion.

There are three different types of angina: stable angina, unstable angina, and variant angina. Stable angina is rhythmic in nature, overexerting the heart on a fairly predictable schedule. Usually this discomfort will cease following rest and/or medication. People who suffer from stable angina are at increased risk for heart attacks.

Unstable angina is a much riskier condition. Those who suffer from this subtype experience pain at unpredictable times. It can occur either while the body is at work or while it is at rest. People who have unstable angina are at immediate risk for a major cardiac event.

The effects of variant angina usually occur when the body is at rest. Medication will often resolve it. This condition is fairly rare, and, like stable angina, those who experience this subtype are at increased risk for a cardiac event.

ANTIANGINALS

Antianginals are those drugs used to treat angina. These medications are typically nitrates, but beta blockers and calcium channel blockers can also be used for the treatment of angina. The usual methods of administering nitrates are **sublingually** (placed under the tongue), orally, and **parenterally**, and may include a sublingual spray or transdermal patches. Those medications that are administered only parenterally have not been included.

Each of the drug categories used to treat angina works in a different way. Nitrates work by dilating the coronary arteries and causing vasodilation throughout the circulatory system. Beta blockers work by decreasing the need for oxygen in the myocardium by decreasing the heart rate. Calcium channel blockers dilate the arteries of the heart allowing greater blood flow to the heart muscle.

antianginals
drug class that is used to prevent the onset of an anginal attack

parenterally
any drug delivery route other than oral

sublingually
under the tongue

Beta-Blocking Agents

Beta-blocking agents work by blocking the effects of adrenaline in certain areas of the body. In doing so, the nerve impulses that control the heart are slowed. Consequently, the heart does not have to work as hard. The body has two types of beta receptors, beta 1 and beta 2. Beta-blocking agents are selective and nonselective depending on which type of beta is blocked.

atenolol

Side Effects: fatigue, weakness, changes in sexual performance
Trade Name: Tenormin
Skin Effects: rashes

carteolol

Side Effects: fatigue, weakness, changes in sexual function
Trade Name: Cartrol
Skin Effects: itching and rashes

labetalol

Side Effects: fatigue, weakness, changes in blood pressure when standing up, changes in sexual performance

Trade Names: Normodyne, Trandate
Skin Effects: itching and rashes

metoprolol

Side Effects: fatigue, weakness, and sexual dysfunction
Trade Names: Lopressor, Toprol-XL
Skin Effects: rashes

nadolol

Side Effects: fatigue, weakness, changes in sexual function
Trade Name: Corgard
Skin Effects: itching and rashes

propranolol

Side Effects: fatigue, weakness, changes in sexual performance
Trade Names: Inderal, Inderal LA
Skin Effects: itching and rashes

Calcium Channel Blockers

Calcium channel blockers relax the blood vessels and increase the blood's oxygen levels, affecting the movement of calcium into the cells of the heart and blood vessels. As a result, blood vessels relax and increase the supply of blood and oxygen to the heart while reducing its workload.

diltiazem

Side Effects: swelling of the arms, legs, hands, and feet
Trade Names: Cardizem, Cardizem LA, Dilacor XR, Tiazac
Skin Effects: dermatitis, **erythema multiforme**, flushing, increased sweating

erythema multiforme
condition characterized by macular eruptions in a patchy formation on the extremities

felodipine

Side Effects: headache, swelling in the arms, legs, hands, and feet
Trade Name: Plendil
Skin Effects: dermatitis, erythema multiforme, flushing, increased sweating

isradipine

Side Effects: swelling in the arms, legs, hands, and feet
Trade Names: DynaCirc, DynaCirc CR

Skin Effects: dermatitis, erythema multiforme, flushing, increased sweating

nicardipine

Side Effects: swelling in the arms, legs, hands, and feet
Trade Names: Cardene, Cardene SR, Cardene IV
Skin Effects: dermatitis, erythema multiforme, flushing, increased sweating, photosensitivity, hives, itching, rash

nifedipine

Side Effects: headache, swelling in the arms, legs, hands, and feet
Trade Names: Adalat, Adalat CC, Procardia, Procardia XL
Skin Effects: flushing, dermatitis, erythema multiforme, increased sweating, photosensitivity, itching, hives, rash.

verapamil

Side Effects: constipation, heartburn, light-headedness, headaches, **lethargy**, flushing, slow heartbeat, and dramatic unusual dreams
Trade Names: Calan, Calan SR, Covera-HS, Isoptin, Isoptin SR, Verelan, Verelan PM
Skin Effects: dermatitis, erythema multiforme, flushing, increased sweating, photosensitivity, **pruritus/urticaria**, rash

lethargy
feelings of excessive sluggishness

pruritus
itching

urticaria
hives

Nitrates

Nitrates work to improve the blood flow to the heart by dilating the coronary arteries. These small arteries supply the heart muscle with blood. When they are restricted, the blood flow is decreased, and heart muscle injury is possible.

isosorbide dinitrate

Side Effects: dizziness, headache, low blood pressure, nausea, restlessness, fainting, fatigue, changes in heartbeat.
Trade Names: Dilatrate-SR, Isorbid, Isordil, Isotrate, Sorbitrate
Skin Effects: flushing of face and neck bluish-colored lips fingernails, or palms of hands, skin rash

isosorbide mononitrate

Side Effects: dizziness, headache, low blood pressure, nausea, restlessness, fainting, fatigue, changes in heartbeat
Trade Name: Imdur, Ismo
Skin Effects: flushing of face and neck, bluish-colored lips, fingernails, or palms of hands, skin rash

nitroglycerin increases the coronary blood flow by dilating the vessels.

Side Effects: dizziness, headache, lower blood pressure, fast heartbeat

Trade Names:

Extended-release capsules: Nitroglyn E-R

Extended-release tablets: Nitrong

Extended release buccal tablets: Nitrogard

Intravenous: Nitro-Bid IV

Translingual Spray: Nitrolingual

Ointment: Nitro-Bid, Nitrol

Sublingual: Nitrostat

Transdermal: Nitrodisc, Nitro-Dur, Transderm-Nitro

Skin Effects: contact dermatitis with the ointment

ANTIARRHYTHMICS

Disturbances in normal heart rhythm, also known as arrhythmias, are common in older adults. In fact, an estimated 4 million Americans are living with arrhythmia. Arrhythmias can occur in a healthy heart and may be of minimal consequence. However, they also may indicate a serious problem and lead to heart disease, stroke, or sudden cardiac death.

Researchers continue to develop new medications that can control arrhythmia. Most common are beta blockers, or beta adrenergic blocking agents. These medications target the adrenaline response of nerve impulses, requiring the heart to not need to work as hard.

Antiarrhythmics are described by class: IA, IB, IC, II, III, IV, and others. Below are some common drugs that are intended to treat arrhythmia.

Class IA

Class IA drugs are used to manage premature ventricular contractions and **ventricular tachycardia**. Many of the drugs used in this category help the heart to be more resistant to abnormal activity.

ventricular tachycardia irregularly rapid heartbeat that is caused by the pumping of the ventricular chambers of the heart

disopyramide

Side Effects: constipation, dry mouth, changes in urination

Trade Names: Norpace, Norpace CR

Skin Effects: skin rash or yellowing of the skin (contact a physician)

moricizine

Side Effects: dizziness, fatigue, headache, nausea
Trade Name: Ethmozine
Skin Effects: none known

procainamide

Side Effects: diarrhea, loss of appetite, dizziness, fever, joint pain or swelling, difficulty breathing, itching, confusion, fever, seizures, asystole, heart block, ventricular arrhythmias, depression
Trade Names: Procanbid, Pronestyl, Pronestyl-SR
Skin Effects: rash

quinidine

Side Effects: diarrhea, stomach pain and cramps, nausea, dizziness or light-headedness, headache, fatigue, weakness, vision changes
Trade Names: Quinaglute Dura-Tabs, Quinidex Extentabs, Quinora
Skin Effects: rash

Class IB

Class IB drugs are used for treatment of arrhythmias associated with **atrioventricular (AV) conduction**. The use of these drugs helps to make the heart more resistant to life-threatening arrhythmias.

fosphenytoin

Side Effects: **ataxia**, double vision, changes in blood pressure, **nystagmus,** gingival hyperplasia, nausea
Trade Names: Cerebyx
Skin Effects: **hypertrichosis**, rashes, exfoliative dermatitis, pruritus

mexiletine slows nerve impulses in the heart, making the heart tissue less sensitive. This drug is used to treat serious arrhythmias.

Side Effects: dizziness, heartburn, nausea and vomiting, anxiety, trembling
Trade Name: Mexitil
Skin Effects: skin rash

tocainide

Side Effects: nausea, diarrhea, vomiting, tremor, headache, changes in mood, changes in vision, drowsiness, hallucinations, restlessness, changes in heartbeat, anorexia

atrioventricular (AV) conduction
component of the cardiac electrical system

ataxia
defective muscle coordination

nystagmus
involuntary and constant movement of the eyeball

hypertrichosis
excessive overgrowth of hair

Trade Name: Tonocard
Skin Effects: rash, sweating, alopecia, flushing

Class IC

These drugs decrease the excitability of the heart, which slows the heart's conduction. These drugs are often used for life-threatening arrhythmias and work on heart muscles to improve the heart's rhythm.

flecainide

Side Effects: blurred vision, dizziness
Trade Name: Tambocor
Possible Skin Effects: skin rash

propafenone

Side Effects: dizziness, heart conduction problems, diarrhea, constipation, vomiting, changes in taste
Trade Name: Rythmol
Skin Effects: skin rash (contact a physician)

Class II

Class II is the category of antiarrhythmic drugs that are beta blockers. These drugs work by blocking the impulses that may cause an irregular heartbeat. Beta blockers also interfere with hormones that could act on the heart such as adrenaline, and in doing so they reduce the blood pressure and the heart rate.

acebutolol

Side Effects: fatigue, weakness, changes in sexual ability
Trade Name: Sectral
Skin Effects: rashes

propranolol

Side Effects: fatigue, weakness, changes in sexual ability
Trade Names: Inderal, Inderal LA
Skin Effects: itching and rashes

sotalol used for the treatment of life-threatening arrhythmias (Betapace) as well as to maintain a normal heartbeat (Betapace AF)
Side Effects: fatigue, weakness, changes in sexual ability

Trade Names: Betapace, Betapace AF
Skin Effects: itching and rashes

Class III

Class III drugs are used in the management of **ventricular arrhythmia** and **atrial flutter.** These drugs work to regulate the heart's rhythm and maintain a **normal sinus rhythm.**

ventricular arrhythmia
irregular heartbeat that has its origin in the ventricular chambers of the heart

atrial flutter
cardiac arrhythmia characterized by a rapid activity of the atrial muscles

normal sinus rhythm
an electrical impulse that regulates the normal heartbeat—usually at a pace of 60–100 beats per minute

peripheral edema
swelling surrounding an injury point, as in around an injection site

amiodarone

Side Effects: dizziness, fatigue, malaise, changes in the cornea of the eye, changes in heartbeat, nausea, vomiting, constipation, anorexia, changes in thyroid function, numbness or tingling in fingers or toes, trembling or shaking of hands, trouble in walking, unusual and uncontrolled movements of the body, weakness of arms, legs, and/or neck
Trade Names: Cordarone, Pacerone
Skin Effects: blue-gray coloring of skin on face, photosensitivity

dofetilide

Side Effects: headache, chest pain, dizziness
Trade Name: Tikosyn
Skin Effects: none known

ibutilide

Side Effects: arrhythmias
Trade Name: Corvert
Skin Effects: none

Class IV

Class IV drugs are used to treat ventricular arrhythmias.

diltiazem

Side Effects: **peripheral edema**
Trade Names: Cardizem, Cardizem LA, Dilacor XR, Tiazac
Skin Effects: dermatitis, erythema multiforme, flushing, increased sweating, photosensitivity, pruritus/urticaria, rash

verapamil

Side Effects: constipation, heartburn, light-headedness, headaches, lethargy, flushing, slow heartbeat, and dramatic unusual dreams

Trade Names: Calan, Cala SR, Covera-HS, Isoptin, Isoptin SR, Verelan, Verelan PM
Skin Effects: dermatitis, erythema multiforme, flushing, increased sweating, photosensitivity, pruritus/urticaria, rash

Others

atropine used in the treatment of arrhythmias

Side Effects: drowsiness, blurred vision, fast heartbeat, dry mouth, changes in urination
Trade Name: AtroPen
Skin Effects: none known

digoxin strengthens the contraction of the heart muscle and slows the heart rate

Side Effects: anorexia, nausea or vomiting, drowsiness, dizziness, fatigue, slowing of heartbeat
Trade Names: Lanoxicaps, Lanoxin
Skin Effects: none noted

Conclusion

Heart disease is the leading killer in the United States today. Whether the disease is high blood pressure, angina, stroke, or one of the other coronary or vascular diseases, medications can help patients live longer, healthier lives. The aesthetician will come into contact with patients taking these medications on a regular basis. It is important to encourage the patients to follow the programs recommended by their physicians. Some of the medications used to treat these problems can cause skin eruptions, rashes, and photosensitivity. If any one of these skin problems occurs, the aesthetician should refer the patients to their physicians for care. Skin problems that are associated with these medications are not within the scope of the aesthetician's care.

REFERENCES

1. http://www.nlm.nih.gov
2. http://www.rxlist.com
3. http://www.drugs.com
4. Deglin, J.H., and Vallerand, A.H. (2007). *Davis's Drug Guide for Nurses.* Philadelphia, PA: F.A. Davis.

5. Michalun, N. (2001). *Milady's Skin Care and Cosmetic Ingredients Dictionary.* Clifton Park: Thomson Delmar Learning.
6. Spratto, G.R., and Woods, A.L. (2005). *2005 PDR Nurse's Drug Handbook.* Clifton Park: Thomson Delmar Learning.
7. http://www.fda.gov

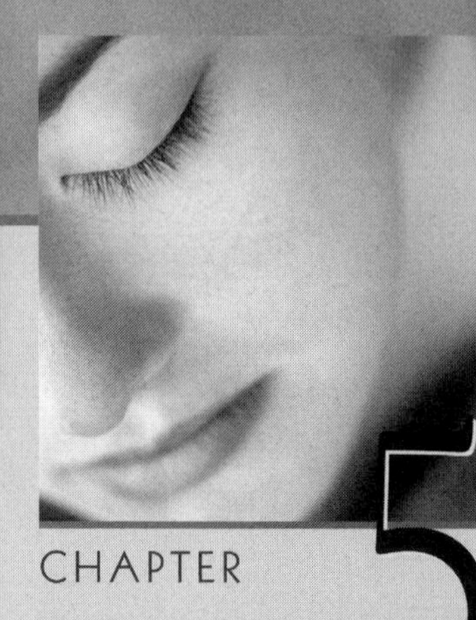

CHAPTER 5

Drugs for Hypertension
Antihypertensives, Diuretics, Beta Blockers, and Calcium Channel Blockers

KEY TERMS

Aldosterone
Diastolic
Essential Hypertension
Hyperkalemia
Hypertension
Hypovolemia
Metabolic Alkalosis
Palpitations
Prehypertension
Primary Hypertension
Sympathetic Outflow
Systolic

LEARNING OBJECTIVES

After completing this chapter, you should be able to:

1. Identify the drug categories used to treat blood pressure problems.
2. Define diastolic blood pressure.
3. Define systolic blood pressure.
4. Define normal blood pressure.

INTRODUCTION

Blood is carried through the body by arteries and veins, and the pump behind this action is the heart. When the blood is pushed against the arteries, it is called the blood pressure. It is the extent of the force against the arteries that determines blood pressure. The blood pressure reading is made up of two numbers: the **systolic** pressure, which is highest when the heart beats, and the **diastolic** pressure, which occurs when the heart is at rest. Both of the numbers are important in determining a normal blood pressure. Blood pressure is written like a fraction with one number over the other. The systolic (when the heart is pumping) is on the top, and the diastolic (when the heart is resting) is on the bottom. For example a normal blood pressure might be 110/75 mm HG. mm Hg, or millimeters of mercury, is how the measurement is taken. The result of a blood pressure reading is communicated by saying the pressure is "110 over 75." Blood pressure normally rises when you get up in the morning, when you are active, or when you have heightened emotion such as anger. Any blood pressure reading below 120/80 is considered normal. If either number or both numbers are elevated, it is considered either **prehypertension** or **hypertension**.

systolic
period in the cycle of the heartbeat in which the heart is contracting

diastolic
period in the cycle of the heartbeat in which the heart is at rest

prehypertension
state of being on the verge of clinic hypertension

hypertension
high blood pressure

essential hypertension
high blood pressure without a known cause

primary hypertension
the first in a series of events in which the affected individual presents with high blood pressure

HYPERTENSION

High blood pressure is called hypertension. Hypertension is determined when one of the numbers in the blood pressure reading is higher than normal. Typically blood pressure that is 120/80 to 140/90 is considered prehypertension. Above 140/90 is considered hypertension. If a physician suspects hypertension, typically he or she will require a blood pressure reading to be taken several times a day, several days in a row. Since the blood pressure can fluctuate, it is important to get a number of readings before determining a diagnosis. Hypertension is referred to as the "silent killer" because the condition does not present with any tangible symptoms that people can detect on their own. However, the effects of the condition can be deadly if not caught and treated. People with untended hypertension are at risk for heart attacks, stroke, and kidney failure.

The symptoms for high blood pressure are rare but occasionally can be attributed to headaches, dizzy spells, and nose bleeds. In a large number of cases the cause is unknown. This type of high blood pressure is called **essential hypertension** or **primary hypertension** and typically develops over years. But some cases of hypertension develop because of underlying causes. Certain diseases such as kidney disease or medications such as birth control pills can create hypertension where the problem previously did not exist. There are certain risk factors that increase the possibility of developing hypertension. These risk factors include age, race, family history, obesity, lack of exercise, tobacco and alcohol use, high sodium intake, and low potassium intake.

ANTIHYPERTENSIVES

The ultimate goal for the treatment of hypertension is to prevent organ damage. There are several subcategories of drugs used to treat hypertension, and they include adrenergics, aldosterane antagonists, ACE inhibitors, angiotensin II receptor antagonists, beta blockers, calcium channel blockers, centrally and peripherally acting antandrenergics, diuretics, and vasodilators. Each of these medications works differently to assist the body in maintaining a normal blood pressure.

Adrenergics

sympathetic outflow
relating to the sympathetic nervous system

aldosterone
adrenal cortex hormone responsible for metabolic regulation

hyperkalemia
abnormally high levels of potassium in the blood

Adrenergics work within the central nervous system to decrease **sympathetic outflow,** reducing blood pressure.

clonidine

Side Effects: drowsiness, dry mouth, withdraw phenomenon
Trade Names: Catapres, Catapres-TTS
Skin Effects: rash and sweating

Aldosterone Antagonists

Aldosterone antagonists block **aldosterone** to lower the blood pressure.

eplerenone

Side Effects: dizziness, fatigue, diarrhea, abdominal pain, flu-like symptoms, **hyperkalemia**
Trade Name: Inspra
Skin Effects: none

(ACE) Inhibitors

These drugs block an enzyme in the body that is necessary to produce a substance that causes blood vessels to tighten. As a result, the vessels relax and blood flows easier. This lowers blood pressure and increases the supply of blood and oxygen to the heart.

benazepril

Side Effects: cough, headache, diarrhea, loss of taste, nausea, changes in the urine
Trade Name: Lotensin
Skin Effects: rashes

captopril

Side Effects: cough, headache, diarrhea, loss of taste, nausea, changes in the urine
Trade Name: Capoten
Skin Effects: rashes

enalapril/enalaprilat

Side Effects: cough, headache, diarrhea, loss of taste, nausea, changes in the urine
Trade Names: Vasotec, Vasotec IV
Skin Effects: rashes

fosinopril

Side Effects: cough, headache, diarrhea, loss of taste, nausea, changes in the urine
Trade Name: Monopril
Skin Effects: rashes

lisinopril

Side Effects: cough, headache, diarrhea, loss of taste, nausea, changes in the urine
Trade Names: Prinivil, Zestril
Skin Effects: rashes

moexipril

Side Effects: cough, headache, diarrhea, loss of taste, nausea, changes in the urine
Trade Name: Univasc
Skin Effects: rashes

perindopril

Side Effects: cough, headache, diarrhea, loss of taste, nausea, changes in the urine
Trade Name: Aceon
Skin Effects: rashes

quinapril

Side Effects: cough, headache, diarrhea, loss of taste, nausea, changes in the urine
Trade Name: Accupril
Skin Effects: rashes

ramipril

Side Effects: cough, headache, diarrhea, loss of taste, nausea, changes in the urine
Trade Name: Altace
Skin Effects: rashes

trandolapril

Side Effects: cough, headache, diarrhea, loss of taste, nausea, changes in the urine
Trade Name: Mavik
Skin Effects: rashes

Antiadrenergics (Centrally Acting)

Antiadrenergics work on the central nervous system to relax the blood vessels and allow the blood to flow more easily, thereby reducing the blood pressure.

guanfacine

Side Effects: confusion, dizziness, drowsiness, fainting, fatigue, headaches, nasal stuffiness, changes in the vision, cough and changes in breathing, chest pain, edema, changes in blood pressure especially when standing up from a sitting position, anorexia, constipation, diarrhea, dry mouth, gas, upset stomach, changes in sexual function, aches and pain in the arms and legs
Trade Name: Tenex
Skin Effects: none known

methyldopa

Side Effects: drowsiness, dizziness, weakness, changes in sexual performance
Trade Name: Aldomet
Skin Effects: itching, rash, and sweating

Antiadrenergics (Peripherally Acting)

Antiadrenergics work peripherally at the nerve endings to lower the blood pressure.

doxazosin

Side Effects: dizziness, drowsiness, headache, confusion, fainting, fatigue, nasal stuffiness, changes in vision, GI symptoms, first dose orthostatic hypotension
Trade Name: Cardura
Skin Effects: flushing, rash, itching, hives

prazosin

Side Effects: dizziness, headache, weakness, change in the blood pressure on the first dose, heart **palpitations**
Trade Name: Minipress
Skin Effects: rash

palpitations the sensation of throbbing

terazosin

Side Effects: nausea, changes in the blood pressure with the first dose
Trade Name: Hytrin
Skin Effects: itching

Angiotensin II Receptor Antagonists

Angiotensin II receptor antagonists work to lower blood pressure and are commonly used by individuals with Type 2 diabetics or those with chronic heart failure.

candesartan

Side Effects: dizziness, fatigue, headache, diarrhea, hyperkalemia, very low blood pressure, drug-induced hepatitis
Trade Name: Atacand
Skin Effects: none noted

eprosartan

Side Effects: dizziness, fatigue, headache, diarrhea, hyperkalemia, very low blood pressure, drug-induced hepatitis
Trade Name: Teveten
Skin Effects: none noted

irbesartan

Side Effects: dizziness, fatigue, headache, diarrhea, hyperkalemia, very low blood pressure, drug-induced hepatitis
Trade Name: Avapro
Skin Effects: none noted

losartan

Side Effects: dizziness, fatigue, headache, diarrhea, hyperkalemia, very low blood pressure, drug-induced hepatitis
Trade Name: Cozaar
Skin Effects: none noted

olmesartan

Side Effects: dizziness, fatigue, headache, diarrhea, hyperkalemia, very low blood pressure, drug-induced hepatitis
Trade Name: Benicar
Skin Effects: none noted

telmisartan

Side Effects: dizziness, fatigue, headache, diarrhea, hyperkalemia, very low blood pressure, drug-induced hepatitis
Trade Name: Micardis
Skin Effects: none noted

valsartan

Side Effects: dizziness, fatigue, headache, diarrhea, hyperkalemia, very low blood pressure, drug-induced hepatitis
Trade Name: Diovan
Skin Effects: none noted

Beta Blockers

Beta blockers work by blocking the effects of adrenaline in certain areas of the body. In doing so, the nerve impulses that control the heart are slowed. Consequently, the heart does not have to work as hard. The body has two types of beta receptors, beta 1 and beta 2. Beta blocking agents are selective and nonselective, depending on which type of beta receptor is blocked.

Nonselective

carteolol

Side Effects: fatigue, weakness, changes in sexual function
Trade Name: Cartrol
Skin Effects: itching and rashes

carvedilol

Side Effects: dizziness, fatigue, weakness, diarrhea, changes in sexual performance, hyperglycemia

Trade Name: Coreg
Skin Effects: itching and rashes

labetalol

Side Effects: fatigue, weakness, changes in blood pressure when standing up, changes in sexual performance
Trade Names: Normodyne, Trandate
Skin Effects: itching and rashes

nadolol

Side Effects: fatigue, weakness, changes in sexual function
Trade Name: Corgard
Skin Effects: itching and rashes

penbutolol

Side Effects: difficulty sleeping, changes in eating (anorexia)
Trade Name: Levatol
Skin Effects: rash and sweating

pindolol

Side Effects: fatigue, weakness, changes in sexual performance
Trade Name: Visken
Skin Effects: itching and rashes

propranolol

Side Effects: fatigue, weakness, changes in sexual performance
Trade Names: Inderal, Inderal LA
Skin Effects: itching and rashes

timolol

Side Effects: fatigue, weakness, changes in sexual performance
Trade Name: Blocadren
Skin Effects: itching, rashes

Selective

acebutolol

Side Effects: fatigue, weakness, changes in sexual performance
Trade Name: Sectral
Skin Effects: rashes

atenolol

Side Effects: fatigue, weakness, changes in sexual performance
Trade Names: Tenormin
Skin Effects: rashes

betaxolol

Side Effects: fatigue, weakness, changes in sexual performance
Trade Name: Kerlone
Skin Effects: rashes

bisoprolol

Side Effects: fatigue, weakness, changes in sexual performance
Trade Name: Zebeta
Skin Effects: rashes

metoprolol

Side Effects: fatigue, weakness, and sexual dysfunction
Trade Names: Lopressor, Toprol-XL
Skin Effects: rashes

Calcium Channel Blockers

Calcium channel blockers relax the blood vessels and increase the blood's oxygen levels, affecting the movement of calcium into the cells of the heart and blood vessels. As a result, blood vessels relax and increase the supply of blood and oxygen to the heart while reducing its workload.

amlodipine

Side Effects: headache, swelling of the arms, legs, hands, and feet
Trade Name: Norvasc
Skin Effects: flushing

diltiazem

Side Effects: swelling of the arms, legs, hands, and feet
Trade Names: Cardizem, Cardizem LA, Dilacor XR, Tiazac
Skin Effects: dermatitis, erythema multiforme, flushing, increased sweating

felodipine

Side Effects: headache, swelling in the arms, legs, hands, and feet
Trade Name: Plendil

Skin Effects: dermatitis, erythema multiforme, flushing, increased sweating

isradipine

Side Effects: swelling in the arms, legs, hands, and feet
Trade Names: DynaCirc, DynaCirc CR
Skin Effects: dermatitis, erythema multiforme, flushing, increased sweating

nicardipine

Side Effects: swelling in the arms, legs, hands, and feet
Trade Names: Cardene, Cardene SR, Cardene IV
Skin Effects: dermatitis, erythema multiforme, flushing, increased sweating, photosensitivity, hives, itching, rash

nifedipine

Side Effects: headache, swelling in the arms, legs, hands, and feet
Trade Names: Adalat, Adalat CC, Procardia, Procardia XL
Skin Effects: flushing, dermatitis, erythema multiforme, increased sweating, photosensitivity, itching, hives, rash.

nisoldipine

Side Effects: headache, swelling in the arms, legs, hands, and feet
Trade Name: Sular
Skin Effects: rash

verapamil

Side Effects: constipation, heartburn, lightheadedness, headaches, lethargy, flushing, slow heartbeat, and dramatic unusual dreams.
Trade Names: Calan, Calan SR, Covera-HS, Isoptin, Isoptin SR, Verelan, Verelan PM
Skin Effects: dermatitis, erythema multiforme, flushing, increased sweating, photosensitivity, pruritus/urticaria, rash

Diuretics

Diuretics reduce the blood volume by decreasing the resistance in the blood vessels, consequently lowering the blood pressure.

chlorothiazide

Side Effects: changes in electrolyte balance in the body, especially potassium

Trade Name: Diuril
Skin Effects: photosensitivity and rashes

chlorthalidone

Side Effects: changes in electrolyte balance in the body, especially potassium
Trade Name: Hygroton
Skin Effects: photosensitivity and rashes

hydrochlorothiazide

Side Effects: changes in electrolyte balance in the body, especially potassium
Trade Names: Esidrex, HydroDIURIL, Oretic
Skin Effects: photosensitivity and rashes

indapamide

Side Effects: changes in potassium balance, change in the levels of uric acid in the blood
Trade Name: Lozol
Skin Effects: photosensitivity, rashes

metolazone

Side Effects: changes in potassium balance, change in the levels of uric acid in the blood
Trade Name: Zaroxolyn
Skin Effects: photosensitivity, rashes

torsemide

Side Effects: dehydration, changes in electrolyte balance, **metabolic alkalosis, hypovolemia**
Trade name: Demadex
Skin Effects: photosensitivity and rashes

metabolic alkalosis
increased alkalines in the body resulting from decreased acids

hypovolemia
abnormally low water levels in the body

Vasodilators

Vasodilators open blood vessels by relaxing the muscle in the vessel walls, causing the blood pressure to drop.

fenoldopam

Side Effects: headache, changes in blood pressure, changes in heart rate, nausea

Trade Name: Corlopam
Skin Effects: flushing and sweating

hydralazine

Side Effects: headache, hypotension, tachycardia, diarrhea, nausea, drug-induced lupus
Trade Name: Apresoline
Skin Effects: rashes

minoxidil

Side Effects: changes in the ECG, changes in the sodium balance, water retention
Trade Name: Loniten
Skin Effects: hypertrichosis, changes in pigment and rashes

nitroprusside

Side Effects: dizziness, headache, stomachache, nausea
Trade Name: Nitopress
Skin Effects: none noted

Conclusion

It is important for those individuals with a family history of hypertension to have a yearly blood pressure taken to ensure the disease has not developed. While it is not within the scope of the aesthetician's license to diagnose or counsel a patient on health issues such as hypertension, it is wise to know the signs of hypertension. If a client presents with one or more of these symptoms, the aesthetician should recommend the care of a physician as critical to the well-being of the patient.

Also, it should be noted that some of the medications found in this category can cause rashes, hives, or itching. The treatment of these skin ailments is not within the scope of the aesthetician's license and should be referred to the physician for treatment. Some of the drugs listed in this chapter cause photosensitivity, and the client should be counseled on the benefits of sunscreen and sun protective clothing when in the sun.

REFERENCES

1. http://www.nlm.nih.gov
2. http://www.rxlist.com
3. http://www.drugs.com

4. Deglin, J.H., and Vallerand, A.H. (2007). *Davis's Drug Guide for Nurses.* Philadelphia, PA: F.A. Davis.
5. Michalun, N. (2001). *Milady's Skin Care and Cosmetic Ingredients Dictionary.* Clifton Park: Thomson Delmar Learning.
6. Spratto, G.R., and Woods, A.L. (2005). *2005 PDR Nurse's Drug Handbook.* Clifton Park: Thomson Delmar Learning.
7. http://www.fda.gov

Antihistamines, Antiasthmatics, and Bronchodilators

CHAPTER 6

KEY TERMS

Anaphylactic Reactions
Antiasthmatics
Antigen
Antihistamines
Asthma
Bronchodilators
Histamine
Immunologic Response
Leukotriene Antagonist
Tachycardia

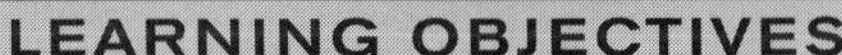

LEARNING OBJECTIVES

After completing this chapter, you should be able to:

1. Define asthma.
2. Discuss hay fever and allergies and the drugs used to treat these problems.
3. Discuss bronchodilators.

antihistamines
any drug that blocks the action of histamine

antiasthmatics
any drug that prevents or limits the severity of the symptoms of an asthma attack

bronchodilators
a group of drugs that are used to reverse acute bronchial constriction

asthma
a chronic condition in which airway restriction results from a triggering event

antigen
any agent that provokes a hypersensitive reaction

immunologic response
process by which the body reacts to a perceived threat and acts to eliminate it or neutralize it

anaphylactic reactions
A form of allergic response to a substance which creates antigen-antibody reactions. This results in severe difficulty in breathing as an initial symptom. See anaphylaxis

histamine
protein in the body that stimulates hypersensitive reactions

INTRODUCTION

Antihistamines, antiasthmatics, and **bronchodilators** are prescribed by physicians to treat a variety of respiratory conditions. The most common of these conditions are allergies and **asthma**, with as many as 1 in 3 Americans suffering from one or both of these conditions. Because the conditions are so common, so are the medications that are used to treat the conditions. As an aesthetician, you will find that the medications listed in this chapter will be among the most common seen in the spa or clinic environment.

ALLERGIES AND SEASONAL HAY FEVER

As many as 45 million Americans suffer from allergies. Hay fever, asthma, and eczema are the most common symptoms of an allergic reaction.

Allergy symptoms surface when the body's immune system responds to a trigger substance as though it were a dangerous invader. This invading substance is called an **antigen** or allergen. The **immunologic response** is accomplished by sending defenders called antibodies to the entry site (most often the nose or skin). The release of chemical mediators, most often histamine, into the bloodstream causes the symptoms that we call allergic reactions.

Symptoms caused by allergic reactions are itching eyes, sneezing, nasal congestion and drainage, and sometimes headache. Some people experience scratchy sore throats, hoarseness, and cough. Other less common symptoms include balance disturbances, swelling in face or throat tissues, skin irritations, respiratory problems, and asthma. **Anaphylactic reactions** are much more serious and may include difficulty breathing, a rash, and a slowed pulse. Anaphylaxis requires immediate medical attention from a qualified medical professional.

ANTIHISTAMINES

As mentioned, **histamine** is a body chemical that is responsible for the symptoms of allergic reaction, including congestion, sneezing, and runny nose. Antihistamines are drugs that block the release of histamine, thereby reducing the allergy symptoms. Most antihistamines produce drowsiness as a side effect when taken. However, newer nonsedating antihistamines, many available only by prescription, do not have this adverse effect. The first few doses may cause sleepiness; subsequent doses are usually less troublesome.

Most antihistamines are available in lower over-the-counter (OTC) dosages, which are sufficient for mild allergy sufferers. Those who experience regular allergies should ask their physicians for a daily allergy medication that is available by prescription.

azatadine relieves the symptoms of hay fever by blocking histamine release

Side Effects: dizziness, fatigue, thickening of bronchial secretions, hypertension, gastric distress, and shifts in menstrual cycles
Trade Name: Optimine
Skin Effects: excessive sweating

brompheniramine an antihistamine that is used to relieve hay fever and allergy symptoms

Side Effects: drowsiness, dry mouth, nose, and throat, upset stomach, headache, chest congestion, diarrhea
Trade Name: Dimetapp
Skin Effects: none

cetirizine an antihistamine that is used to relieve hay fever and allergy symptoms by blocking histamine release

Side Effects: dizziness, drowsiness, fatigue, dry mouth
Trade Name: Zyrtec
Skin Effects: dry skin

clemastine an antihistamine that is used to relieve hay fever and allergy symptoms

Side Effects: drowsiness, dry mouth, nose, and throat, dizziness, upset stomach, chest congestion, headache
Trade Name: Tavist
Skin Effects: none

cyproheptadine relief of seasonal allergies and colds by blocking histamine release

Side Effects: drowsiness, excitation, blurred vision, dry mouth
Trade Name: Periactin
Skin Effects: photosensitivity, rashes

desloratadine relief of seasonal allergies and colds by blocking histamine release

Side Effects: drowsiness, dry mouth
Trade Name: Clarinex
Skin Effects: none

diphenhydramine an antihistamine, relieves red, irritated, itchy, and watery eyes; sneezing; and runny nose caused by hay fever, allergies, and the common cold.

Side Effects: dry mouth, nose, and throat, drowsiness, upset stomach, chest congestion, headache
Trade Name: Benadryl
Skin Effects: none

fexofenadine an antihistamine that is used to relieve hay fever and allergy symptoms

Side Effects: headache, dizziness, drowsiness, back pain, cough
Trade Name: Allegra
Skin Effects: none

loratadine nondrowsy relief of seasonal allergies and colds by blocking histamine release

Side Effects: confusion, excitation, blurred vision, dry mouth
Trade Names: Alavert, Claritin, Clear-Atadine
Skin Effects: photosensitivity, rash

promethazine relief of seasonal allergies and colds by blocking histamine release

Side effects: sedation, disorientation, dizziness, blurred vision, constipation, dry mouth
Trade Name: Phenergan
Skin Effects: photosensitivity, skin rash

ASTHMA

Asthma is a disease of the respiratory system in which the airways become blocked or narrowed, causing breathing difficulty. This chronic disease affects nearly 20 million Americans. Asthma is commonly divided into two types: allergic asthma (which is caused from allergens) and nonallergic asthma (which is most often caused by physical activity). There is still much research that needs to be done to fully understand how to prevent, treat, and cure asthma, but, with proper management, people can live healthy and active lives.

ANTIASTHMATICS

Antiasthmatics are drugs that treat asthma symptoms from a multitude of attack modes. They are further classified according to short term and long term symptom management. Long term asthma relief targets the causes and triggers of asthma attacks, whereas short term asthma relief is meant to target relief of the symptoms of asthma attacks once they occur.

cromolyn mast cell stabilizer used for long term control of activity-induced bronchospasms

Side Effects: irritation of the nose, throat, and trachea, and unpleasant taste
Trade Names: Intal and NasalCrom
Skin Effects: erythema, rash, and hives

epinephrine relieves reversible airway constriction associated with asthma or severe allergic reaction

Side Effects: nervousness, tremors, restlessness, angina, arrhythmias, hypertension, tachycardia
Trade Names: Adrenalin, EpiPen, Primatene
Skin Effects: flushing, erythema

nedocromil mast cell stabilizer used for long term control of activity-induced bronchospasms

Side Effects: irritation of the nose, throat, and trachea, and unpleasant taste
Trade Name: Tilade
Skin Effects: erythema, rash, and hives

zafirlukast **leukotriene antagonist** that acts to control asthma related symptoms.

Side Effects: headache, dizziness, diarrhea, nausea
Trade Name: Accolate
Skin Effects: none

leukotriene antagonist agent that acts as an inhibitor of leukotrienes, a chemical mediator of inflammation

Other Drugs Used to Treat Asthma

Aside from the conventional treatments specifically intended to treat asthma, other treatments can overlap with treatments for other conditions. The following medications are explained in greater detail in other parts of this text, yet warrant discussion as they relate to asthma in this section.

Bronchodilators: See Below

albuterol
formoterol

levalbuterol
metaproterenol
pirbuterol
salmeterol
terbutaline

Corticosteroids: See Chapter 15

beclomethasone
betamethasone
budesonide
cortisone
dexamethasone
flunisolide
fluticasone
hydrocortisone
methylprednisolone
prednisolone
prednisone
triamcinolone

BRONCHODILATORS

Bronchodilators are drugs that relieve airway constrictions caused by a number of conditions including asthma. They relieve symptoms quickly and are therefore often referred to as short term relief drugs. These drugs may be administered by inhalation, by oral means, or by means of injections. Most of these medications are delivered via inhalation.

It is commonly thought that inhaled medicines are strong medicines and a person gets dependent on inhalers. But this is false. In fact, inhaled medications work fast and are quite safe because they are available in much lower doses and have fewer side effects.

albuterol used to control and limit airway constriction caused by asthma

Side Effects: nervousness, restlessness, tremors, palpitations, chest pain
Trade Names: Proventil, Ventolin, Volmax
Skin Effects: none

epinephrine relieves reversible airway constriction associated with asthma or severe allergic reaction

Side Effects: nervousness, tremors, restlessness, angina, arrhythmias, hypertension, **tachycardia**
Trade Names: Adrenalin, AsthmaHaler Mist, AsthmaNefrin, EpiPen, microNefrin, Nephron, Primatene
Skin Effects: flushing, erythema

tachycardia
a faster than normal heart rate

formoterol long term control mechanism for asthma symptoms that limits bronchospasms

Side Effects: dizziness, fatigue, muscle cramps, dry mouth, tremors
Trade Name: Foradil
Skin Effects: flushing, erythema

levalbuterol short term control mechanism for asthma symptoms by limiting bronchospasms

Side Effects: dizziness, nervousness, anxiety
Trade Name: Xopenex
Skin Effects: flushing, erythema

montelukast management of chronic asthma symptoms as well as seasonal allergies

Side Effects: fatigue, headache, weakness, cough, abdominal pain
Trade Name: Singulair
Skin Effects: rash

pirbuterol quick relief of airway constriction resulting from asthma or similar diseases

Side Effects: nervousness, restlessness, tremors, insomnia, arrhythmias
Trade Name: Maxair
Skin Effects: flushing, erythema

salmeterol long term maintenance of airway constriction due to asthma related bronchospasm and exercise related asthma attacks

Side Effects: headache, diarrhea, stomach cramps, cough
Trade Name: Serevent
Skin Effects: flushing, erythema

terbutaline short and long term management of airway constriction from asthma related causes

Side Effects: nervousness, restlessness, tremor, insomnia, arrhythmias, nausea, vomiting
Trade Names: Brethaire, Brethine, Bricanyl
Skin Effects: flushing, erythema

theophylline long term maintenance of asthma symptoms, including airway constriction

Side effects: anxiety, tachycardia, nausea, vomiting
Trade Names: Elixophyllin, Quibron-T, Theobid, Theo-Dur, Uniphyl
Skin Effects: none

zafirlukast long term management of asthma and asthma related symptoms

Side Effects: headache, dizziness, weakness, abdominal pain, diarrhea, nausea, vomiting
Trade Name: Accolate
Skin Effects: none

Conclusion

Antihistamines, antiasthmatics, and bronchodilators are used to treat a wide range of respiratory conditions including asthma and allergies. Because of the high rate of frequency of these conditions, these are among the most common medications you will encounter as an aesthetician. While some of these medications will have no skin effects, many will, which you should consider when planning a skin treatment regime for your clients.

As mentioned before, it is important to have a complete Health History Sheet from your clients. Cross referencing these medications with the information provided to you by the client will ensure the best treatment for your client. Also mentioned, which cannot be stressed enough, it is outside your scope of practice to make any recommendations regarding medication to your clients. If you suspect that any of the medications the client may be taking is responsible for his or her skin care concerns, you should refer the patient to a qualified physician.

REFERENCES

1. http://www.nlm.nih.gov
2. http://www.rxlist.com
3. http://www.drugs.com
4. Deglin, J. H., and Vallerand, A. H. (2007). *Davis's Drug Guide for Nurses.* Philadelphia, PA: F. A. Davis.
5. Michalun, N. (2001). *Milady's Skin Care and Cosmetic Ingredients Dictionary.* Clifton Park: Thomson Delmar Learning.
6. Spratto, G. R., and Woods, A. L. (2005). *2005 PDR Nurse's Drug Handbook.* Clifton Park: Thomson Delmar Learning.
7. http://www.fda.gov

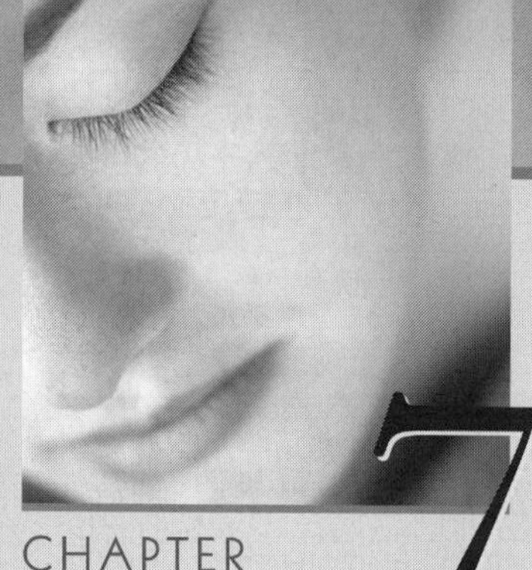

CHAPTER 7

Drugs Used to Treat Gastrointestinal and Urinary Disorders

KEY TERMS

5-HT_3 Antagonists
Antacids
Anticholinergics
Antiemetics
Antispasmodics
Antiulcer Drugs
Chronic Acid Reflux Disease
Chronic Metabolic Acidosis
Erosive Esophagitis
Hyperacidity
Hypomagnesemia
Irritable Bowel Syndrome
Neurogenic Bladder
Nocturia
Overactive Bladder
Peptic Ulcer
Phenothiazines
Proton Pump Inhibitors

LEARNING OBJECTIVES

After completing this chapter, you should be able to:

1. Discuss the reasons for nausea and vomiting and the products used to treat this problem.
2. Discuss ulcers.

INTRODUCTION

Among some of the more common conditions that patients seek medical attention for are those associated with disruptions in the normal functioning of the gastrointestinal tract and urinary functions. These include everything from frequent heartburn to urinary incontinence to **peptic ulcers**. Most of the conditions are rather benign, but are often painful and inconvenient.

Yet, because the conditions are so common, the medications that are used to treat them are equally common. Therefore many of the medications listed below will appear often on Health History Sheets.

The medications discussed in this chapter are available both by prescription and as over-the-counter (OTC) products. When investigating your clients' health histories, be sure to ask them what OTC medications they take on a regular basis, as many people will not include this information.

peptic ulcer
a wearing down of normal tissue of the stomach and esophagus, resulting in frequent stomach pain, especially after eating

anticholinergics
drug class that acts to limit spasms and cramping, particularly of the digestive and urinary tracts

antispasmodics
drugs used to treat motion sickness, nausea, vomiting or spasms and muscle cramps of the intestinal tract or bladder

irritable bowel syndrome
condition of unknown etiology characterized by disturbances of normal bowel function

ANTICHOLINERGICS

The **anticholinergics**, also called **antispasmodics**, are part of a drug category that includes drugs used to treat cramps (spasms) of the stomach, intestines, and bladder. Such cramping results in upset stomach, nausea, vomiting, and a variety of bladder conditions.

Anticholinergics are also used in certain surgical and emergency procedures. In surgery, some are given by injection before anesthesia to help relax the patient and to decrease secretions, such as saliva. During anesthesia and surgery, they are often used to help keep the heartbeat normal and to prevent nauseous side effects of the anesthetic. Anticholinergics can also be used for painful menstruation, for runny noses, and for the prevention of urination during sleep. As you can see, this category has a variety of uses.

atropine management of **irritable bowel syndrome** and peptic ulcers

Side Effects: drowsiness, blurred vision, tachycardia, dry mouth, difficulty urinating
Trade Names: no brand name
Skin Effects: flushing and decreased sweating

darifenacin regulates bladder and urinary urges and frequency

Side Effects: constipation, dry mouth, nausea
Trade Name: Enablex
Skin Effects: none

dicyclomine management of irritable bowel syndrome

Side Effects: drowsiness, constipation, heartburn
Trade Name: Bentyl
Skin Effects: decreased sweating

hyoscyamine relief for a variety of gastric symptoms including gastric secretions, spastic bladder, and abdominal cramping

Side Effects: blurred vision, nausea, dizziness, nervousness, dry mouth
Trade Names: Anaspaz, Cystospaz, Levsinex, Levsin, Levbid
Skin Effects: urticaria and decreased sweating

neurogenic bladder
improper bladder functioning resulting in overactivity or underactivity of normal urinary function

nocturia
excessive and frequent urination at night

overactive bladder
condition characterized by abnormally high levels of bladder activity resulting in frequent need to urinate

oxybutynin treats **neurogenic bladder** conditions related to urgency, **nocturia**, incontinence, and **overactive bladder**

Side Effects: dizziness, fatigue, blurred vision constipation, bloating
Trade Name: Ditropan
Skin Effects: urticaria and decreased sweating

solifenacin treats symptoms associated with overactive bladder

Side Effects: constipation, dry mouth, nausea
Trade Name: VESIcare
Skin Effects: none

tolterodine treats symptoms associated with overactive bladder

Side Effects: headache, dizziness, dry mouth
Trade Names: Detrol and Detrol LA
Skin Effects: none

ANTIDIARRHEALS

As one can decipher by the name, antidiarrheals are drugs that are used to prevent or relieve the symptoms of diarrhea. Antidiarrheal drugs operate according to one of two separate mechanisms. They either thicken the stool or regulate intestinal spasms.

The remedies that operate by thickening the stool usually contain clay or other substances that absorb the bacteria or toxins that cause diarrhea. Stool thickeners are safe due to the fact that they do not go into the blood. However, long term usage can be problematic because the flora needed for normal functioning is absorbed as well.

The other mode of operation regulates or reduces intestinal spasms that result in diarrhea. Loperamide (the active ingredient in products such as Imodium A-D and Pepto Diarrhea Control) is an example of this type of remedy. Some products contain both thickening and antispasmodic ingredients.

bismuth subsalicylate used to treat diarrhea, upset stomach, and indigestion in adults

Side Effects: side effects are rare when taken as directed, but overdosing symptoms include anxiety, hearing loss, confusion, constipation, diarrhea, slurred speech, dizziness, drowsiness, breathing difficulties, headache, increased sweating, thirst, depression, muscle spasms, muscle weakness, nausea, ringing in ears, stomach pain, trembling, vision problems
Trade Names: Bismatrol, Bismatrol Extra Strength, Pepto-Bismol, Pepto-Bismol Easy-to-Swallow Caplets, Pepto-Bismol Maximum Strength
Skin Effects: none

difenoxin/atropine adjunctive therapy for diarrhea

Side Effects: dizziness, headache, constipation, dry mouth, nausea
Trade Name: Motofen
Skin Effects: flushing

diphenoxylate/atropine adjunctive therapy for diarrhea

Side Effects: dizziness, headache, constipation, dry mouth, nausea
Trade Names: Lomotil, Lonox
Skin Effects: flushing

kaolin/pectin a clay-like powder believed to work by attracting and holding onto the bacteria or germ that may be causing the diarrhea

Side Effect: constipation
Trade Name: Kaopectate
Skin Effects: none

loperamide treatment of acute diarrhea and diarrhea associated with inflammatory bowel syndrome

Side Effects: drowsiness, constipation, dry mouth, nausea
Trade Names: Diar-aid Caplets, Imodium, Imodium A-D, Kaopectate II Caplets, Maalox Anti-Diarreheal Caplets, Neo-Diaral, Pepto Diarrhea Control
Skin Effects: none

ANTIEMETICS

Nausea and vomiting occur for many reasons. The most common causes are motion sickness or self-limited illnesses that last a few hours to a few days. However, nausea can also be caused by more serious conditions that may require the care of a physician. For most, nausea is a temporary, and bothersome, condition. Yet it is easily treated with many over-the-counter (OTC) and prescription drugs.

An antiemetic is a drug that is effective against vomiting and nausea. **Antiemetics** are typically used to treat motion sickness and the side effects of opioid analgesics. Often, they are prescribed to prevent chemotherapy-related nausea in cancer patients. There are several different types of antiemetics, which are classified according to their mode of operation.

antiemetics
any drug that prevents or limits the severity of the symptoms of nausea and vomiting

5-HT$_3$ antagonists
antienemics that are selective serotonin inhibitors, which inhibit the binding of serotonin to 5-HT$_3$ receptors

5-HT$_3$ Antagonists

The **5-HT$_3$ antagonists** are selective serotonin inhibitors, which inhibit the binding of serotonin to 5-HT$_3$ receptors, hence the name. The resulting processes are complicated, yet the net result is a reduction in the symptoms of nausea and vomiting. The 5-HT$_3$ antagonists are most often prescribed for cancer patients undergoing chemotherapy; however, they are also prescribed for people prone to prolonged nausea or motion sickness. For instance, people who suffer from motion sickness and who plan to fly a long distance may request a prescription from their physicians.

dolasetron prevents nausea and vomiting

Side Effects: headache, dizziness, diarrhea
Trade Name: Anzemet
Skin Effects: pruritis

granisetron prevents nausea and vomiting, particularly in chemotherapy and postoperative patients

Side Effects: headache, anxiety, constipation
Trade Name: Kytril
Skin Effects: none

ondansetron prevents nausea and vomiting, particularly in chemotherapy and postoperative patients

Side Effects: headache, constipation, diarrhea, dry mouth
Trade Name: Zofran
Skin Effects: none

Phenothiazines

Phenothiazines are most often used to treat serious mental and emotional disorders, including schizophrenia and other psychotic disorders. However, they can also be used to control some of the severest cases of nausea and vomiting.

phenothiazines
type of drug used to treat schizophrenic disorders

chloropromazine used to treat nausea and vomiting as well as intractable hiccups

Side Effects: blurred vision, dry eyes, hypotension, constipation, dry mouth
Trade Name: Thorazine
Skin Effects: photosensitivity, pigment changes, rashes

prochlorperazine treatment of nausea and vomiting

Side Effects: blurred vision, dry eyes, constipation, dry mouth
Trade Name: Compazine
Skin Effects: photosensitivity, pigment changes, rashes

promethazine treatment of nausea, vomiting, and motion sickness

Side Effects: confusion, disorientation, sedation
Trade Name: Phenergan
Skin Effects: photosensitivity, rashes

Other Antiemetic Drugs

aprepitant treats acute vomiting and nausea

Side Effects: dizziness, fatigue, diarrhea
Trade Name: Emend
Skin Effects: none

dimenhydrinate treats nausea, vomiting, motion sickness, and vertigo

Side Effects: drowsiness, anorexia
Trade Name: Dramamine
Skin Effects: photosensitivity

meclizine treats nausea associated with motion sickness

Side Effects: drowsiness, blurred vision, dry mouth
Trade Names: Antrizine, Dramamine Less Drowsy Formula, Meni-D, Vergon
Skin Effects: none

scopolamine prevention of nausea and vomiting associated with motion sickness

Side Effects: drowsiness, blurred vision, tachycardia, dry mouth, difficulty urinating
Trade Names: Isopto Hyoscine, Transderm Scop
Skin Effects: none

ANTIULCER DRUGS

Anyone who suffers from peptic ulcers knows that they are painful and persistent conditions that can have a great effect on the quality of life for those who suffer from them. A peptic ulcer is a hole in the gut lining of the stomach, duodenum, or esophagus. A peptic ulcer of the stomach is called a gastric ulcer; of the duodenum, a duodenal ulcer; and of the esophagus, an esophageal ulcer. An ulcer occurs when the lining of these organs is corroded by the acidic digestive juices that are secreted by the stomach cells. Left untreated, ulcers can have some serious consequences, which may require surgery to repair.

Medications that are used to relieve the symptoms of ulcers are called **antiulcer drugs**. This is a drug category that is further subcategorized according to the modes of operation. The drugs include **antacids**, H2 Histamine Inhibitors, and **Proton Pump Inhibitors**. Some are available only with a prescription, while others are available in over-the-counter (OTC) dosages.

antiulcer drugs
any drug that prevents or limits the severity of the symptoms of peptic ulcers

antacid
any agent that neutralizes stomach acid

Proton Pump Inhibitors
any antiulcer agent that restricts the acid production in the stomach

hyperacidity
condition in which the body produces too much acid

Antacids

Antacids are taken by mouth to relieve heartburn, sour stomach, or acid indigestion. They work by neutralizing excess stomach acid. Some antacid combinations also contain simethicone, which may relieve the symptoms of excess gas. Antacids alone or in combination with simethicone may also be used to treat the symptoms of stomach or duodenal ulcers. These medicines are generally available without a prescription.

aluminum hydroxide treatment of duodenal and gastric ulcers, **hyperacidity**, and acid reflux

Side Effects: constipation
Trade Names: AlternaGEL, Alu-Cap, Aluminet, Alu-Tab, Amphojel, Basalgel, Dialume
Skin Effects: none

magnesium hydroxide/ aluminum hydroxide treatment of **hypomagnesemia** and hyperacidity

Side Effects: diarrhea, constipation
Trade Names: Maalox and Mylanta
Skin Effects: flushing and sweating

Proton Pump Inhibitors

esomeprazole used to treat **chronic acid reflux disease**

Side Effects: headache, constipation, dry mouth, nausea
Trade Names: Nexium
Skin Effects: none

lansoprazole used to treat chronic acid reflux disease in association with duodenal or gastric ulcers, **erosive esophagitis**, and heartburn

Side Effects: dizziness, headache, diarrhea
Trade Name: Prevacid
Skin Effects: rash

omeprazole used to treat chronic acid reflux disease in association with duodenal or gastric ulcers, erosive esophagitis, and heartburn

Side Effects: dizziness, drowsiness, abdominal pain, diarrhea, nausea, vomiting
Trade Names: Prilosec, Prilosec OTC
Skin Effects: rash and pruritus

rabeprazole used to treat chronic acid reflux disease in association with duodenal or gastric ulcers, erosive esophagitis, and heartburn

Side Effects: dizziness, headache, constipation, diarrhea, nausea
Trade Name: Aciphex
Skin Effects: photosensitivity and rash

HISTAMINE H2 ANTAGONIST

Studies have shown that the protein histamine (see Chapter 6) stimulates gastric acid secretion, which is responsible for ulcer irritation. Histamine antagonists are drugs designed to restrict histamine on gastric cells, hence reducing acid output. While H2 blockers are effective in reducing the symptoms of ulcers, they do not cure the underlying conditions. Therefore, ulcers frequently return when H2 blockers are stopped.

hypomagnesemia
abnormally low levels of magnesium in the blood accompanied by muscle irritability

chronic acid reflux disease
recurrent condition characterized by stomach acids slipping into the esophagus, resulting in a burning sensation in the chest. Also known as GERD

erosive esophagitis
condition characterized by the eroding of the esophagus; most commonly caused by chronic acid reflux disease

cimetidine short term relief of duodenal and gastric ulcers

Side Effects: confusion, dizziness, drowsiness, diarrhea, nausea
Trade Names: Tagamet, Tagamet HB
Skin Effects: none

famotidine short term relief of duodenal and gastric ulcers

Side Effects: confusion, dizziness, drowsiness, diarrhea, nausea
Trade Names: Maximum Strength Pepcid, Pepcid AC, Pepcid RPD
Skin Effects: none

nizatidine short term relief of duodenal and gastric ulcers

Side Effects: confusion, dizziness, drowsiness, diarrhea, nausea
Trade Names: Axid, Axid AR
Skin Effects: none

raniditine short term relief of duodenal and gastric ulcers

Side Effects: confusion, dizziness, drowsiness, diarrhea, nausea
Trade Names: Zantac, Zantac 75, Zantac 150
Skin Effects: none

ranitidine bismuth citrate short term relief of duodenal and gastric ulcers

Side Effects: confusion, dizziness, drowsiness, diarrhea, nausea
Trade Name: Tritec
Skin Effects: none

MINERALS USED TO TREAT ULCERS

Aside from the antiulcer drugs whose purpose is specific, many minerals that our bodies require normally can be used to treat the symptoms of peptic ulcers.

sodium bicarbonate antacid

Side Effects: metabolic alkalosis, water retention, flatulence, gastric distention
Trade Names: Baking Soda, Bell-Ans, Citrocarbonate, Neut, Soda Mint
Skin Effects: none

sodium citrate and citric acid treats **chronic metabolic acidosis**

Side Effects: diarrhea
Trade Names: Bicitra, Oracit, Shohl's Solution
Skin Effects: none

chronic metabolic acidosis
condition characterized by the body having an abnormally low pH level

Calcium Salts

calcium acetate treats hyperacidity and heartburn

Side Effects: arrhythmias, constipation, nausea, vomiting, phlebitis
Trade Names: Calphron, PhosLo
Skin Effects: none

calcium carbonate treats hyperacidity and heartburn; also used as a calcium supplement

Side Effects: upset stomach, vomiting, stomach pain, belching, constipation, dry mouth, increased urination, loss of appetite, metallic taste
Trade Names: Alka-Mints, Amitone, BioCal, Calcarb, CalciChew, Calciday, Calcilac, Calci-Mix, Cal-Plus, Caltrate, Chooz, Dicarbosil, Equilet, Liqui-Cal, Maalox Antacid Caplets, Os-Cal, Rolaids Calcium Rich, Surpass, Tums, Tums E-X
Skin Effects: none

calcium citrate treats hyperacidity and heartburn; also used as a calcium supplement

Side Effects: arrhythmias, constipation, nausea, vomiting, phlebitis
Trade Names: Cal-Citrate 250, Citrical, Citrical Liquitabs
Skin Effects: none

calcium gluconate treats hyperacidity and heartburn; also used as a calcium supplement

Side Effects: arrhythmias, constipation, nausea, vomiting, phlebitis
Trade Name: Kalcinate
Skin Effects: none

calcium lactate treats hyperacidity and heartburn; also used as a calcium supplement

Side Effects: arrhythmias, constipation, nausea, vomiting, phlebitis
Trade Name: Cal-LAC
Skin Effects: none

tricalcium phosphate treats hyperacidity and heartburn; also used as a calcium supplement

Side Effects: arrhythmias, constipation, nausea, vomiting, phlebitis
Trade Name: Posture
Skin Effects: none

Magnesium Salts

magnesium chloride treats/prevents hypomagnesia as well as used as an antacid

Side Effects: diarrhea
Trade Names: Chloromag, Slow-Mag
Skin Effects: flushing and sweating

magnesium citrate treats/prevents hypomagnesia as well as used as an antacid and as a laxative

Side Effects: diarrhea
Trade Names: Citrate of Magnesia, Citroma
Skin Effects: flushing and sweating

magnesium gluconate treats/prevents hypomagnesia as well as used as an antacid

Side Effects: diarrhea
Trade Names: Almoate, Magtrate, Magonate
Skin Effects: flushing and sweating

magnesium hydroxide treats/prevents hypomagnesia as well as used as an antacid

Side Effects: diarrhea
Trade Names: Dulcolax Magnesia Tablets, Phillips' Magnesia Tablets, Phillips' Milk of Magnesia
Skin Effects: flushing and sweating

magnesium oxide treats/prevents hypomagnesia as well as used as an antacid

Side Effects: diarrhea
Trade Names: Mag-Ox 400, Maox, Uro-Mag
Skin Effects: flushing and sweating

Conclusion

As mentioned, gastrointestinal and urinary disorders are among the most common conditions that affect the aging population. By the time most individuals reach the age of 60, they will have experienced one or more of the conditions mentioned in the previous pages. As someone who provides skin care services, you will assist many clients who come to your workplace having these conditions. Although you cannot treat these consequences of aging, it is important to know whether your clients are taking these medications. While most are benign, some do cause rashes and changes in pigmentation, which may be responsible for the client's skin concerns.

It is important to have a complete health history, including the use of over-the-counter (OTC) medications. Many of the drugs contained within this chapter are available OTC. Whether the medications used by your client are used OTC or under the advisement of a doctor, it is not within your scope of practice to offer any advice concerning the usage of these drugs. If you suspect that the usage of any drug is responsible for the skin condition, refer the client to the prescribing physician for further investigation.

REFERENCES

1. http://www.fda.gov/cder/consumerinfo/OTClabel.htm
2. http://www.nlm.nih.gov
3. http://www.rxlist.com
4. http://www.drugs.com
5. Deglin, J. H., & Vallerand, A. H. (2007). *Davis's Drug Guide for Nurses.* Philadelphia, PA: F. A. Davis.
6. Michalun, N. (2001). *Milady's Skin Care and Cosmetic Ingredients Dictionary*. Clifton Park: Thomson Delmar Learning.
7. Spratto, G. R., & Woods, A. L. (2005). *2005 PDR Nurse's Drug Handbook.* Clifton Park: Thomson Delmar Learning.
8. http://www.fda.gov

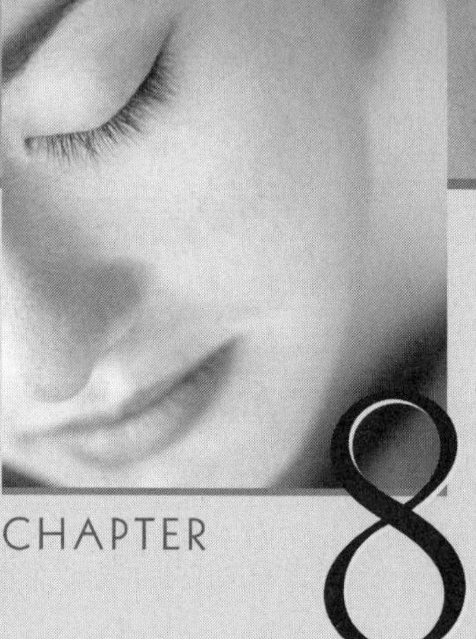

CHAPTER 8

Pyschotropic Drugs

KEY TERMS

Antianxiety Drugs
Anticonvulsants
Antidepressants
Antipsychotics
Ataxia
Barbiturates
Benzodiazepines
Bipolar Disorder
Central Nervous System Stimulants
Clamminess
Depression
Diplopia
Dysmorphia
Dysmorphic
Dyspepsia
Dysthymia
Epilepsy
Extrapyramidal
Generalized Anxiety Disorder (GAD)
Gingival Hypoplasia
Hallucinations
Hydantoin Anticonvulsants
Hypotension
Jaundice
Major Depression
Mental Illness
Monoamine Oxidase Inhibitors (MAOIs)
Neuroleptic Drugs
Norepinephrine
Nystagmus
Obsessive-Compulsive Disorder
Oligohydrosis
Paresthesia
Phenothiazines
Phobias
Physical Dependence
Post-Traumatic Stress Disorder
Psychological Dependence
Psychosis
Schizophrenia
Select Serotonin Reuptake Inhibitors
Serotonin
Social Phobias
Tricyclics
Trigeminal Neuralgia
Valproates Anticonvulsants
Vertigo

LEARNING OBJECTIVES

After completing this chapter, you should be able to:

1. Define the different types of mental illnesses.
2. Identify the medications that are used to treat mental illnesses.
3. Explain the side effects of the drugs used to treat mental illnesses.
4. Explain the skin effects of the drugs used to treat mental illnesses.

INTRODUCTION

Mental illnesses are some of the more common disorders to afflict Americans. In fact, at any one given point, roughly 10 percent of the population suffers from a **mental illness**.[1] However, many cases go undiagnosed and untreated because many people do not realize that the feelings they have are symptomatic of a condition, let alone a condition that can be treated with medications.

mental illness
umbrella term for any condition that results in a measurable dysfunction of mental or psychotic functioning

depression
condition characterized by low mood, loss of interest, loss of energy, changes in weight, changes in appetite, changes in sleep patterns, fatigue, inability to concentrate, feelings of low self-worth, and possibly thoughts of suicide

A mental illness is considered to be a condition that produces disturbances in an individual's thoughts, emotions, or behavior. Scientists believe that these conditions are due to an imbalance of chemicals in the brain. Most pharmacologic remedies are targeted toward these chemicals with the goal of being able to achieve a healthy balance that will result in the stabilization of the afflicted individual's mood or behavior.

Mental illness encompasses a wide variety of treatable conditions that have an equally wide range of symptoms. Mild **depression** on one end of the spectrum causes an individual to feel sad and lethargic, while psychotic disorders, such as multiple personality disorder, can render an individual incapable of performing even the most perfunctory of tasks. Regardless of the specific disorder, they all have one characteristic in common: they interfere with a person's ability to live a normal life. People with severe mental illnesses cannot hold a job, relate to other individuals, or cope with the ordinary events of life. Different medications are used to treat various mental conditions; however, some overlap exists.

Currently, there are about 50 different medications that are approved to treat mental conditions. Some of the side effects of these medications can make taking them a difficult decision, but it comes down to weighing the benefits of the medication versus the side effects. If a patient experiences undesirable side effects, then he or she often consults with the prescribing physician and switches to an alternative medication that might not have the undesired side effects.

ANXIETY-RELATED CONDITIONS

Everybody experiences normal levels of anxiety in their lives. But anxiety in its most extreme cases can render an individual paranoid, alone, and often housebound. Collectively, anxiety disorders are the most common mental illnesses in the United States. Over 20 million individuals have one of the several diseases that make up this disease category.[2] Fortunately, drugs are available to alleviate the suffering of the affected

[1] http://www.nimh.nih.gov
[2] http://www.nimh.nih.gov

individuals by easing the fear and paranoia while improving the quality of life.

Under the general category of anxiety disorders, there are five specific disorders that all have their own unique characteristics and symptoms. Those disorders are panic disorder, **obsessive-compulsive disorder,** **post-traumatic stress disorder**, **phobias**, and **generalized anxiety disorder**.

obsessive-compulsive disorder (OCD)
anxiety disorder characterized by perpetual and excessive thoughts and activities that interfere with the normal functioning of the affected individual

post-traumatic stress disorder
anxiety condition that is the result of stress brought on by a traumatic event

phobias
anxiety condition characterized by unwarranted fear such that it interferes with the normal functioning of the affected individual

generalized anxiety disorder (GAD)
condition characterized by unspecific or unwarranted anxiety

Panic Disorder

Panic disorder is a condition in which the affected individual suffers from panic attacks that are accompanied by physical symptoms, which include heart palpitations, light-headedness, and sweating. Emotionally, they are riddled to their core about a perceived threat. There is often no warning before the onset of an attack, and the individual is in a constant state of low-grade anxiety anticipating the next attack. The panic attacks can happen anytime, even while the individual is asleep.

Women are more likely than men to experience this condition. The onset of the condition usually occurs in late adolescence and can be progressive.

Obsessive-Compulsive Disorder

Obsessive-compulsive disorder (OCD) is a condition characterized by two main components: obsessive behavior and compulsive behavior. The obsessive component involves the uncontrollable need to constantly be fixated on or concerned about an item or perceived threat. This is accompanied by an uncontrollable urge to engage in a ritual to combat the threat. One example would be an irrational fear of dirt or bacteria, which causes the individual to wash his or her hands or body until it is raw. The affected individual garners no pleasure or relief by performing these rituals, which, left unchecked, can become a major disruption in the individual's life.

The onset of this condition is variant. It occurs in children as often as it does in adults. It is a persistent condition that does not resolve itself very easily, though treatments are becoming available that have yielded some positive results.

Post-Traumatic Stress Disorder

Post-traumatic stress disorder (PTSD) is an anxiety disorder that is brought on by the brain's inability to process the repercussions of a traumatic, frightening, or emotionally charged event. People who suffer from

PTSD are riddled with unwelcome images, memories, or dreams of the triggering event. Often they take extra precautions to avoid places, people, or events that remind them of the triggering event. Most people associate post-traumatic stress as being an immediate product of the event, but, in reality, the symptoms can take months, even years, to fully manifest themselves. Left untreated, they can morph into more complex mental disorders.

Phobias

Some people view phobias from an indifferent perspective—they tend to view them with a sense of humor. However, some people are so limited by their fears that they are virtually debilitated. Depending on what the fear is, affected individuals may be so fearful that they can alienate everyone with whom they come in contact.

Phobias are subcategorized into two separate types: **social phobias** and specific phobias. Social phobias are fears of people and social situations. Those who have social phobias are constantly wondering what other people think about them and how other people perceive them, their appearance, and their words. They spend so much time considering these issues that they are unable to enjoy themselves, communicate, or perform many of the tasks required in social situations.

social phobias
fear of public places or interacting with other people, which results in the need to avoid that which interferes with normal functioning

Specific phobias relate to a fear of a specific item, event, or situation. Comparatively speaking, specific phobias are much easier to cope with, and many people are able to hide their fears for prolonged periods of time. They tend to know that their fears are irrational; however, they are subject to paralyzing fear when confronted with the object of

Table 8-1 Events That Can Lead to PTSD
Rape or sexual abuse
Physical abuse
Victim of a violent crime
Airplane or automobile accident
Natural disaster
War
Life-threatening illness or event
Witness to any of the aforementioned events

their fear. The specific item determines the individual's ability to function. For example, an individual with a fear of darkness or water has more of a challenge to overcome the phobia than an individual who fears snakes.

Generalized Anxiety Disorder

Generalized anxiety disorder (GAD) is a disease that creeps up on the people who suffer from it. Once its effects become known, the individual who suffers from GAD becomes ineffectual in the daily tasks associated with living.

Those living with this condition experience severe and exaggerated fears and tension about some of the more mundane aspects of life. They are concerned, to the point of paranoia, that some of these normal events of their lives are an attempt to derail them or hurt them. This paranoia can reach into all aspects of their lives and cause them considerable setbacks with regards to their individual pursuits.

Antianxiety Drugs

Effective treatments for each of the anxiety disorders have been developed through research. In general, two types of treatment are available for an anxiety disorder—medication and specific types of psychotherapy (sometimes called "talk therapy"). Both approaches can be effective for most disorders. The choice of one or the other, or both, depends on the patient's and the doctor's preference, as well as on the particular anxiety disorder.

The medications used to treat anxiety-related conditions are referred to as **antianxiety drugs**. They operate on the central nervous system to sedate and regulate impulses that result in anxiety-related symptoms such as increased heartbeat and paranoia. They are prescribed for either short term or long term management of the symptoms, either to prevent them or to negate them once they begin.

antianxiety drugs
any drug that prevents or limits the severity of the symptoms of an anxiety disorder

benzodiazepines
group of drugs with a sedative effect; predominantly used to treat anxiety and sleep disorders

physical dependence
chemical dependence in which the body thinks it needs a substance in order to function

Benzodiazepines

Benzodiazepines are a type of central nervous system (CNS) depressants, meaning that they slow down the nervous system. Most benzodiazepines are used to relieve anxiety, but only for the most extreme cases of diagnosed conditions. However, if used regularly, they usually are not effective for more than a few weeks.

Benzodiazepines may be habit-forming (causing mental or **physical dependence**), so care must be taken in the use of these medications.

alprazolam manages and relieves panic attacks

Side Effects: dizziness, drowsiness, lethargy, diarrhea, nausea, vomiting, physical dependence
Trade Names: Xanax, Xanax XR
Skin Effects: rashes

chlordiazepoxide relief from anxiety and chemical withdrawal

Side Effects: dizziness, drowsiness, constipation, diarrhea, nausea, vomiting
Trade Name: Librium
Skin Effects: rashes

diazepam anxiety management, sedation, and chemical withdrawal

Side Effects: dizziness, drowsiness, lethargy, constipation, nausea, vomiting, phlebitis, physical dependence
Trade Name: Valium
Skin Effects: rashes

lorazepam manages anxiety and insomnia

Side Effects: dizziness, drowsiness, lethargy, blurred vision, constipation, nausea, vomiting, physical dependence
Trade Name: Ativan
Skin Effects: rashes

midazolam manages anxiety, sedation

Side Effects: phlebitis, agitation, drowsiness, blurred vision, nausea, vomiting
Trade Name: Versed
Skin Effects: rashes

oxazepam treatment of anxiety and alcohol withdrawal

Side Effects: dizziness, drowsiness, impaired memory, slurred speech, constipation, diarrhea, physical dependence
Trade Name: Serax
Skin Effects: rashes

buspirone treatment for anxiety

Side Effects: dizziness, drowsiness, excitement, fatigue, headache, insomnia, weakness, blurred vision, nasal congestion, sore throat, chest pain, palpitations, tachycardia, nausea, myalgia, loss of coordination, numbness, tremors, **clamminess**, sweating

clamminess
sensation of the skin feeling cool to the touch

Trade Name: BuSpar
Skin Effects: rashes

doxepin treatment of anxiety

Side Effects: fatigue, sedation, blurred vision, **hypotension**, constipation, dry mouth
Trade Names: Sinequan, Zonalon
Skin Effects: photosensitivity and rashes

hydroxyzine pamoate management of anxiety

Side Effects: drowsiness, dry mouth, bitter taste, constipation, nausea
Trade Name: Vistaril
Skin Effects: flushing

hydroxyzine HCL management of anxiety

Side Effects: drowsiness, dry mouth, bitter taste, constipation, nausea
Trade Name: Atarax
Skin Effects: flushing

paroxetine hydrochloride management of depression, anxiety, panic disorder, obsessive-compulsive disorder, generalized anxiety disorder, post-traumatic stress disorder, premenstrual **dysmorphic** disorder

Side Effects: anxiety, dizziness, drowsiness, headache, insomnia, weakness, constipation, dry mouth, nausea, ejaculatory disturbance, decreased libido, tremors
Trade Names: Paxil, Paxil CR
Skin Effects: sweating, photosensitivity, pruritus, rashes

venlafaxine treatment of **major depression**, generalized anxiety disorder, social anxiety disorder

Side Effects: seizures, abnormal dreams, anxiety, dizziness, headache, insomnia, nervousness, weakness, rhinitis, changes in vision, abdominal pain, changes in taste, loss of appetite (often resulting in weight loss), constipation, diarrhea, dry mouth, **dyspepsia**, nausea, vomiting, sexual dysfunction, **paresthesia**, chills
Trade Names: Effexor, Effexor XR
Skin Effects: ecchymoses, pruritus, photosensitivity, rashes

ANTICONVULSANTS

Anticonvulsants are a type of drug used to reduce the frequency and severity of seizures resulting from a variety of conditions. The most common of

hypotension
low blood pressure

dysmorphic
abnormally formed

major depression
severest type of depression characterized by severe and frequent instances of low mood, loss of interest, loss of energy, changes in weight, changes in appetite, changes in sleep patterns, fatigue, inability to concentrate, feelings of low self-worth, and possibly thoughts of suicide

dyspepsia
symptomatic condition characterized by abnormal or painful digestion

paresthesia
sensation of numbness and prickling, often called "pins and needles"

anticonvulsants
any drug that prevents or limits the severity of spastic activity resulting from certain neurological conditions

these conditions is **epilepsy**. Epilepsy is a neurological condition with unknown etiology. It might be the result of genetics, or it might be the result of a head injury. Epilepsy is not the only cause for seizures. Other situations, such as chemical withdrawal or low blood sugar, can also result in a patient seizing.

There are several different types of anticonvulsant medications that act to depress the central nervous system in a variety of manners. The exact pharmacology of their actions is beyond the scope of this text. The different types of anticonvulsants include **barbiturates**, benzodiazepines (see above), hydantoins, and valproates.

Barbiturates

Barbiturates are central nervous system depressants. They act on the brain and the CNS to produce effects that may be helpful or harmful. This depends on the individual patient's condition and response and the amount of medicine taken.

Barbiturates are often used as anticonvulsants to help control seizures in certain disorders or diseases, such as epilepsy. Barbiturates may also be used for other conditions as determined by a doctor. If too much of a barbiturate is used, it may become habit-forming.

phenobarbital anticonvulsant used to treat seizures in children

Side Effects: hangover, drowsiness, constipation, diarrhea, dry mouth, dyspepsia, nausea, vomiting, physical and **psychological dependence**
Trade Name: Luminal
Skin Effects: photosensitivity, urticaria, rashes

Hydantoins

Hydantoin anticonvulsants are most commonly used in the treatment of seizures associated with epilepsy. Some hydantoins, such as phenytoin, are also indicated for use as skeletal muscle relaxants and in the treatment of severe nerve pain, as in **trigeminal neuralgia.**

fosphenytoin short term management of seizures

Side Effects: **ataxia**, **diplopia**, **nystagmus**, hypotension, **gingival hypoplasia**, nausea,
Trade Name: Cerebyx
Skin Effects: hypertrichosis, rashes, exfoliative dermatitis, pruritus

epilepsy
neurologic condition characterized by sudden seizures

barbiturates
addictive central nervous system depressants

psychological dependence
type of chemical dependence characterized by the affected individuals thinking they need a substance for normal functioning

hydantoin anticonvulsants
drugs that are most commonly used in the treatment of seizures associated with epilepsy

trigeminal neuralgia
nerve pain along the nerves of the face

ataxia
defective muscle coordination

diplopia
seeing double

gingival hypoplasia
underdevelopment of the gum tissue

nystagmus
horizontal twitching of the eyes

phenytoin short term management of seizures

Side Effects: ataxia, diplopia, nystagmus, hypotension, gingival hypoplasia, nausea
Trade Name: Dilantin
Skin Effects: hypertrichosis, rashes, exfoliative dermatitis, pruritus

Valproates

valproates anticonvulsants
drugs that are meant to limit the frequency and severity of spastic activity

bipolar disorder
mental condition characterized by periods of high activity and then severe depression

Valproates anticonvulsants are most commonly used in the treatment of seizures associated with epilepsy. Some valproates, such as Depakote, are also indicated for use as skeletal muscle relaxants and in the treatment of **bipolar disorder**.

divalproex sodium management of seizures and manic episodes associated with bipolar disorder

Side Effects: confusion, dizziness, headache, indigestion, nausea, vomiting
Trade Names: Depakote, Depakote ER
Skin Effects: rashes

valproate sodium management of seizures

Side Effects: confusion, dizziness, headache, indigestion, nausea, vomiting
Trade Name: Depacon
Skin Effects: rashes

valproic acid management of seizures

Side Effects: confusion, dizziness, headache, indigestion, nausea, vomiting
Trade Name: Depakene
Skin Effects: rashes

Other Anticonvulsant Drugs

acetazolamide seizure management

Side Effects: depression, fatigue, weakness, loss of appetite (resulting in weight loss), metallic taste in mouth, hyperchloremic acidosis, anemia, paresthesia
Trade Name: Diamox
Skin Effects: rashes

carbamazepine management of seizures, treatment of bipolar disorder

Side Effects: ataxia, drowsiness, blurred vision, hypotension
Trade Names: Tegretol, Tegretol XR
Skin Effects: photosensitivity, rash, urticaria

gabapentin adjunct treatment for partial seizures

Side Effects: confusion, depression, drowsiness, hostility, **vertigo**, changes in vision, ataxia
Trade Name: Neurontin
Skin Effects: none

vertigo
sensation of moving through space or of having objects float independently around; often synonymous with dizziness

lamotrigine adjunct treatment of seizures for individuals with epilepsy and Lennox-Gastaut Syndrome, and maintenance of bipolar disorder

Side Effects: ataxia, dizziness, headache, nausea, vomiting
Trade Name: Lamictal
Skin Effects: photosensitivity and rash

levetiracetam manages partial seizures

Side Effects: dizziness, weakness
Trade Name: Keppra
Skin Effects: none

oxcarbazepine manages partial seizures in adults

Side Effects: dizziness, vertigo, drowsiness, headache, changes in vision, diplopia, nystagmus, abdominal pain, nausea, ataxia, coordination problems, tremors
Trade Name: Trileptal
Skin Effects: acne, rash, urticaria

pregabalin manages partial seizures in adults

Side Effects: dizziness, drowsiness, dry mouth
Trade Name: Lyrica
Skin Effects: edema

tiagabine adjunct treatment of seizures

Side Effects: dizziness, drowsiness, weakness
Trade Name: Gabatril
Skin Effects: alopecia, dry skin, rash, sweating

topiramate manages seizures, particularly seizures arising from Lennox-Gastaut Syndrome

Side Effects: dizziness, drowsiness, fatigue, reduced memory and concentration, problem with motor skills, slurred speech, abnormal vision, diplopia, nystagmus, dry mouth, weight loss, ataxia, paresthesia
Trade Name: Topamax
Skin Effects: **oligohydrosis**

oligohydrosis
condition characterized by excessive low water levels in the body

dysthymia
chronic and mild depression often occurring from secondary antagonists (i.e., side effect from medication)

antidepressants
any drug that prevents or limits the severity of the symptoms of depression

zonisamide manages partial seizures in adults

Side Effects: drowsiness
Trade Name: Zonegran
Skin Effects: oligohydrosis

benzodiazepines see above

DEPRESSION

A temporary sense of depression will affect most Americans at least once over the course of their lifetime. While people use the word "depressed" very loosely, clinical depression is defined as a condition that affects the mood, behaviors, and bodies of an individual over an extended period of time. People who are clinically depressed cannot merely "pull it together" and shake it off. They need treatment, with or without medications, to remedy the condition.

There are three different types of depression. The first and most common type is called mild depression, or **dysthymia**. People who suffer from dysthymia usually have persistent depressive symptoms that prevent them from feeling or functioning their best. They are also likely to experience a major depressive event over the course of their lives. Since the symptoms are mild, many people do not recognize that they are clinically depressed until they have a major depressive event, and hindsight allows them to see that they have been unhappy for a prolonged period of time. Treatment of dysthymia is short term treatment with talk therapy or medicinal **antidepressants**.

The second type of depression is major depression. Major depression encompasses a severe expression of depressive symptoms (see Table 8.3),

Table 8-2 Benzodiazepines Used to Treat Convulsive Disorders
Clonazepam
Clorazepate
Diazepam

Table 8-3 Symptoms of Depression
Persistent sad, empty, or anxious feelings
Pessimism
Feelings of guilt or lack of self-worth
Loss of interest in things that were once enjoyable
Loss of energy
Difficulty concentrating
Sleep pattern disturbances (sleeping too much or insomnia)
Eating pattern disturbances (weight gain or loss)
Thoughts of suicide
Irritability
Chronic body pains (joints, muscles, headaches)

such that it poses a major intrusion on the affected individuals ability to function. Treatment for major depression is more long term, involving talk therapy, antidepressants, or a combination of both.

The third type of depression is bipolar disorder. Because the symptoms and medications used to treat bipolar disorder are different from the milder versions of depression, we discuss it later in this chapter.

Researchers have compiled a great amount of data about depression and the demographics of those who suffer from it. They have surmised that certain groups within the population at large are more vulnerable to depression. For instance, women are twice as likely to receive a diagnosis of depression than men. There are several suspected reasons for this, among them the hormonal factors associated with menstruation, pregnancy, and menopause. While men are less likely to be diagnosed, it does not mean that the occurrence is less. Men are less likely to seek treatment than women and are less likely to admit feeling depressed. This is evidenced by the fact that men have a suicide rate that is four times the suicide rate for women.

Similarly, individuals with a family history of depression are more likely to have a depressive episode than those who do not. This can be seen in the prevalence of recent childhood depression diagnoses. Likewise, the elderly and those who live in poor economic conditions have high occurrence rates, though a smaller rate of seeking treatment. While these individuals are more likely to experience a depressive event, anyone, regardless of sex, age, race, or class, can experience a depressive event.

Treatment of Depression

Collectively, the medications that are used to treat depression are called antidepressants. Antidepressants were first developed in the 1950s and have been used regularly since then. The exact mechanisms under which they operate are not entirely clear. However, it is known that they affect neurotransmitters, particularly dopamine, **serotonin**, and **norepinephrine**.

There are three major categories of antidepressants. They are **tricyclics** (TCAs), **select serotonin reuptake inhibitors** (SSRIs), and **monoamine oxidase inhibitors** (MAOIs).

Tricyclics were the first antidepressants to become available. They are powerful drugs that increase the brain's supply of norepinephrine and serotonin. The downside to TCAs is that the side effects can often be severe and are not tolerated by some. Also, the failure rate is around 30 percent, a statistic that is common to all antidepressants.

Select serotonin reuptake inhibitors are best for individuals who are in the early stages of less severe depressive states. They are newer and accompanied by less severe side effects. While they are generally better tolerated, their success rate is not any greater than TCAs, about 60–70 percent. In addition, they are expensive. The good news is that because the patents for many of these drugs will expire in coming years, the costs should go down.

Monoamine oxidase inhibitors (MAOIs), like TCAs, affect the levels of norepinephrine and serotonin, as well as the dopamine levels. An enzyme in our brains, called monoamine oxidase, destroys neurotransmitters before they have an opportunity to convey their messages to the receptors. MAOIs inhibit this enzyme, allowing a buildup of neurotransmitters.

While antidepressants have proven to be effective and have helped millions of people, finding the right one is a complicated process. Whether it is the failure of a particular drug to achieve positive outcomes or the inability of the patient to tolerate the drug, many will have to switch medications several times before finding one that works effectively and can be tolerated.

serotonin
neurotransmitter that is thought to be a major contributor to many mental illnesses including depression, anxiety disorders, and personality disorders

norepinephrine
hormone produced in the adrenal medulla that acts as a vasoconstrictor

tricyclics (TCAs)
the most commonly prescribed type of antidepressants used to treat the milder cases of depression or anxiety

select serotonin reuptake inhibitors (SSRIs)
type of antidepressant that allows for more productive use of the neurotransmitter serotonin

monoamine oxidase inhibitors (MAOIs)
drug treatment for depression. The exact mode of their action is not quite understood

Selective Serotonin Reuptake Inhibitors

citalopram used to treat depression. It is a SSRI or selective serotonin reuptake inhibitor.

Side Effects: apathy, confusion, drowsiness, insomnia, weakness, abdominal pain, anorexia, diarrhea, dry mouth, dyspepsia, flatulence, increased saliva, nausea, tremor
Trade Name: Celexa
Skin Effects: increased sweating

duloxetine hydrochloride used to treat depression

Side Effects: Fatigue, drowsiness, insomnia, decreased appetite, constipation, dry mouth, nausea, dysuria
Trade Name: Cymbalta
Skin Effects: changes in sweating

escitalopram used to treat depression and generalized anxiety disorder

Side Effects: insomnia, diarrhea, nausea, constipation, dry mouth, increased appetite
Trade Name: Lexapro
Skin Effects: increased sweating

fluoxetine used to treat depression. It is also used to treat obsessive-compulsive disorder, eating disorders, and panic attacks. Under the brand name of Sarafem the drug is used to treat PMS. Fluoxetine is an SSRI.

Side Effects: Anxiety, drowsiness, headache, insomnia, nervousness, diarrhea, changes in sexual performance, tremor
Trade Name: Sarafem, Prozac
Skin Effects: excessive sweating, itching

fluvoxamine used to treat obsessive-compulsive disorder. It is an SSRI.

Side Effects: Dizziness, drowsiness, headache, insomnia, nervousness, weakness, constipation, diarrhea, dry mouth, upset stomach, nausea
Trade Name: Luvox
Skin Effects: sweating, skin rash, hives

paroxetine used to treat panic attacks, depression, social anxiety disorders, and obsessive-compulsive disorders. It is also used to treat premenstrual, dysphoric disorder. It is a SSRI.

Side Effects: Anxiety, dizziness, drowsiness, headache, insomnia, weakness, constipation, diarrhea, dry mouth, nausea, changes in sexual function, tremor
Trade Name: Paxil
Skin Effects: sweating, sun sensitivity

sertraline used to treat depression, obsessive-compulsive disorder, panic attacks, post-traumatic stress disorder, and disorders associated with social interaction. It is also used to treat PMS. It is a SSRI medication.

Side Effects: Dizziness, drowsiness, fatigue, headache, insomnia, diarrhea, dry mouth, nausea, changes in sexual function, tremor
Trade Name: Zoloft
Skin Effects: increased sweating

Tetracyclic and Tricyclic Antidepressants

amitriptyline used for the relief of endogenous depression

Side Effects: Lethargy, changes in vision, dry eyes, dry mouth, constipation, low blood pressure
Trade Names: Elavil, Endep, Etrafon
Skin Effects: increased sweating. photosensitivity

amoxapine used to treat depression

Side Effects: stomachache, sleepiness, weakness, excitement, increased anxiety, changes in sleep patterns including nightmares, dry mouth, changes in weight, changes in appetite
Trade Name: Asendin
Skin Effects: sun sensitivity

buspirone used to treat increased anxiety, generally for a short period of time

Side Effects: stomachache or sour stomach, vomiting, constipation, diarrhea, changes in sleep, drowsiness or fatigue, anxiety, agitation, headache, dry mouth, depression, light-headedness, weakness, numbness, muscles
Trade Name: Buspar
Skin Effects: skin rashes, itching.

desipramine hydrochloride used to treat depression, this is a tricyclic antidepressant. This drug should be used with caution in children.

Side Effects: Fatigue, sleepiness, blurred vision, dry eye, dry mouth, constipation, low blood pressure
Trade Name: Norpramin
Skin Effects: photosensitivity

doxepin hydrochloride this drug is one of the dibenzoxepin tricyclic compounds used to treat depression

Side Effects: Fatigue, sleepiness, blurred vision, low blood pressure, constipation, dry mouth

Trade Names: Adapin, Sinequan
Skin Effects: Skin rash, photosensitization

imipramine used to treat depression

Side Effects: sleepiness, fatigue, blurred vision, dry mouth, dry eyes, constipation, low blood pressure.
Trade Name: Tofranil
Skin Effects: photosensitivity

mirtazapine used to treat depression

Side Effects: Sleepiness, constipation, dry mouth, changes in appetite, weight gain.
Trade Name: Remeron
Skin Effects: Sensitivity to touch, rash, itching

nortriptyline used to treat depression

Side Effects: Fatigue, sleepiness, blurred vision, dry eyes, dry mouth, low blood pressure, constipation
Trade Names: Pamelor, Aventyl
Skin Effects: sun sensitivity.

Monoamine Oxidase Inhibitors

When other antidepressants do not work, some people find relief from an older class of medications known as MAO inhibitors. Monoamine oxidase inhibitors (MAOIs) were the first type of antidepressant to be used, starting in the 1950s. MAOIs relieve depression by preventing the enzyme monoamine oxidase from breaking down the neurotransmitters norepinephrine, serotonin, and dopamine in the brain. Higher levels of these chemicals result, and mood is boosted. These drugs are used much less frequently now, because they can have dangerous side effects.

For the small number of people for whom MAOIs are the best treatment, it is necessary to avoid certain foods that contain high levels of tyramine, such as many cheeses, wines, and pickles, as well as medications such as decongestants. The interaction of tyramine with MAOIs can bring on a hypertensive crisis, a sharp increase in blood pressure that can lead to a stroke. The doctor should furnish a complete list of prohibited foods that the patient should carry at all times. Other forms of antidepressants require no food restrictions.

Some people do find these medications to be lifesaving. For these people MAOIs can be the best treatment. As long as they are vigilant about their diet, they can get real relief from their depression.

phenelzine used to treat depression. It is a MAOI.

Side Effects: changes in weight, changes in appetite, dry mouth, changes in sleep including strange or unpleasant dreams. sour stomach, drowsiness, weakness or tiredness, anxiety, or agitation.
Trade Name: Nardil
Skin Effects: sun sensitivity.

tranylcypromine used to treat depression. It is a MAOI.

Side Effects: sour stomach, changes in appetite, changes in weight, dry mouth, drowsiness, changes in sleep with possible unpleasant dreams, agitation, excitement, weakness, or tiredness. constipation, changes in urination, changes in sexual performance or sexual desires, blurry vision.
Trade Name: Parnate
Skin Effects: sun sensitivity, increased sweating.

Other Antidepressant Drugs

bupropion used to treat depression, increases certain brain activities

Side Effects: sour stomach, vomiting, weight loss, constipation, changes in sleep, drowsiness, restlessness, agitation, anxiety, dry mouth, headache, dizziness, and tremors.
Trade Name: Wellbutrin
Skin Effects: excessive sweating

nefazodone used for the treatment of depression

Side Effects: diarrhea, constipation, nausea, vomiting, heartburn, dry mouth, dizziness, sleepiness and changes in appetite.
Trade Name: Serzone
Skin Effects: sun sensitivity, rashes

trazodone used for the management of depression. It is a serotonin modulator.

Side Effects: Sleepiness, low blood pressure, dry mouth
Trade Name: Desyrel
Skin Effects: sweating, rash

venlafaxine treatment of major depression, generalized anxiety disorder, social anxiety disorder

Side Effects: seizures, abnormal dreams, anxiety, dizziness, headache, insomnia, nervousness, weakness, rhinitis, changes in vision, abdominal pain, changes in taste, loss of appetite (often resulting in weight loss), constipation, diarrhea, dry mouth, dyspepsia, nausea, vomiting, sexual dysfunction, paresthesia, chills

Trade Names: Effexor, Effexor XR

Skin Effects: ecchymoses, pruritus, photosensitivity, rashes

PSYCHOTIC DISORDERS

Psychotic disorders are among the most dangerous types of mental disorders, not only to the individuals themselves, but for those around them as well. The distortion of thought processes and reality can be so extreme that an affected individual loses sight of what is and is not, and what is right and what is wrong. The good news, however, is that psychotic disorders by definition are only temporary. The major symptom of these disorders is **psychosis**, or delusions and **hallucinations.** Delusions are false beliefs that significantly hinder a person's ability to function, for example, believing that people are trying to hurt you when there is no evidence of this, or believing that you are somebody else. Hallucinations are false perceptions. They can be visual (seeing things that are not there), auditory (hearing things that are not there), olfactory (smelling things that are not there), tactile (feeling sensations on your skin that are not really there, such as the feeling of bugs crawling on you), or taste.

The cause of this disorder is typically an extremely stressful event or trauma.

Psychotic disorders are usually treated with talk therapies, and often medication. The medicines that are used to treat psychotic disorders belong to the family of medicines known as thioxanthenes, also called **antipsychotics**.

psychosis
most extreme cases of mental disturbance in which the affected individual has partially or totally lost touch with reality, either permanently or temporarily

hallucinations
symptom in which an individual sees or hears things which are not actually there

antipsychotics
any drug that prevents or limits the severity of the symptoms of psychosis

neuroleptic drugs
any medication that has side effects that resemble symptoms of neurologic diseases

Antipsychotic Drugs

The term **antipsychotic** is applied to a group of drugs used to treat **psychosis**. Common conditions for which antipsychotics might be used include schizophrenia, mania, and delusional disorder, although antipsychotics might be used to counter psychosis associated with a wide range of other diagnoses. Antipsychotics also have some effects as mood stabilizers, leading to their frequent use in treating mood disorder (particularly bipolar disorder) even when no signs of psychosis are present. Some antipsychotics are used to treat Tourette's syndrome.

Antipsychotics are also referred to as **neuroleptic drugs**, or simply neuroleptics. The word "neuroleptic" is derived from Greek. "Neuro" refers to the nerves and "lept" means "to take hold of." Thus, the word means "taking hold of one's nerves," which implies their role in mood stabilization.

Phenothiazines

phenothiazines
type of drug used to treat schizophrenic disorders

schizophrenia
personality disorder characterized by a disassociation from social experience and limited social range

extrapyramidal
existing outside of the pyramidal tracts of the central nervous system

Phenothiazines are used to treat serious mental and emotional disorders, including **schizophrenia** and other psychotic disorders. Some are used also to control agitation in certain patients, severe nausea and vomiting, severe hiccups, and moderate to severe pain in some hospitalized patients.

Phenothiazines may cause unwanted, unattractive, and uncontrolled face or body movements that may not go away after one has stopped taking the medicine. They may also cause other serious unwanted effects.

chlorpromazine used to treat psychotic disorders. It also has other uses such as the treatment of nausea and vomiting, behavior problems in children, and the management of hiccups.

Side Effects: dry mouth, drowsiness. Low blood pressure, blurry vision
Trade Name: Thorazine
Skin Effects: skin discolorations such as yellow-brown to gray and purple.

fluphenazine used to treat schizophrenia and symptoms such as hallucinations. It is an antipsychotic drug.

Side Effects: **extrapyramidal** reactions
Trade Names: Permitil, Prolixin
Skin Effects: sun sensitivity.

prochlorperazine used to treat a variety of conditions including anxiety, psychoses, and nausea and vomiting

Side Effects: extrapyramidal reactions, blurred vision, dry eyes, constipation, dry mouth
Trade Name: Compazine
Skin Effects: photosensitivity, pigment changes, rashes

thioridazine used to treat schizophrenic patients. It is usually used once other treatments have failed. It is an antipsychotic drug, but it has side effects that could endanger the life of the patient.

Side Effects: Sleepiness, blurry vision, dry eyes, changes in blood pressure, constipation, dry mouth
Trade Name: Mellaril
Skin Effects: Photosensitivity, rashes, changes in pigment.

trifluoperazine used to treat schizophrenia and associated symptoms such as hallucinations. It is also used for anxiety in patients who need short term relief.

Side Effects: sleepiness, vertigo, changes in vision, GI upset, and other GI symptoms such as nausea, vomiting, diarrhea, constipation, weight gain. agitation, headache
Trade Name: Stelazine
Skin Effects: Pigment changes, rashes, photosensitivity

Other Antipsychotic Drugs

aripiprazole used to treat schizophrenia. It is an antipsychotic medication.

Side Effects: changes in sleep, nervousness, lethargy, light-headedness, changes in weight, constipation, uncontrollable tremorcoughing, runny nose, headache, itchy eyes, earaches, loss of appetite, and restlessness.
Trade Name: Abilify
Skin Effects: dry skin and rashes.

benzodiazepines see above

clozapine used to treat schizophrenia. It is used as a second line drug after other drugs have not been effective. It is an antipsychotic.

Side Effects: diarrhea, constipation, restlessness, headache, or lethargy.

Table 8-4 Benzodiazepines Used as Sedatives/Hypnotics
Chlordiazepoxide
Clorazepate
Diazepam
Flurazepam
Lorazepam
Midazolam
Oxazepam
Temazepam
Triazolam

jaundice
yellowing of the skin most offer caused by improper liver functioning

Trade Name: Clozaril
Skin Effects: **jaundice,** abnormal bruising

haloperidol used to treat different types of mental and emotional conditions. It is also used to treat the symptoms of Tourette's disorder.

Side Effects: changes in vision, changes in menstrual cycle, breast swelling and unusual breast secretions, dry mouth, constipation, weight gain. Changes in sexual performance, lethargy, nausea, and vomiting.
Trade Name: Haldol
Skin Effects: sun sensitivity.

olanzapine used to treat schizophrenia. This drug is an antipsychotic.

Side Effects: constipation and diarrhea, drowsiness, agitation, headache, sleepiness, weakness, orthostatic hypotension, dry mouth, tremor, weight gain
Trade Name: Zyprexa
Skin Effects: photosenstivity

quetiapine used to treat hallucinations and other psychotic symptoms and disorders

Side Effects: vertigo, faintness, GI symptoms such as stomach pain, constipation, and weight gain, which could be significant.
Trade Name: Seroquel
Skin Effects: rash

risperidone used to treat schizophrenia and suicidal tendencies

Side Effects: GI upset and symptoms such as weight gain, GI pain, constipation, diarrhea, heartburn, changes in sleep with bad dreams, sleepiness, vertigo, excitement, agitation, changes in sexual performance or desires, changes in the quality of the menstrual period. Cold or flu-like symptoms such as runny nose, cough, sore throat, muscle aches and pains. Changes in urination.
Trade Name: Risperdal
Skin Effects: dry skin that changes color

ziprasidone used to manage schizophrenia

Side Effects: sleepiness constipation, diarrhea, changes in appetite, changes in weight. muscle aches and pains, cough, sneezes, runny nose. Agitation
Trade Name: Geodon
Skin Effects: rash, hives, and sweating

CENTRAL NERVOUS SYSTEM STIMULANTS

Whereas central nervous system depressants slow down the functions of the CNS in people suffering from anxiety disorders, **central nervous system stimulants** increase the activity for people suffering from conditions such as narcolepsy.

central nervous system stimulants
any drug that increases central nervous system activity

amphetamine mixtures used to treat both narcolepsy and attention deficit/hyperactivity disorder (ADHD)

Side Effects: hyperactivity, insomnia, restlessness, tremors, heart palpitations, tachycardia, decreased appetite (resulting in weight loss), psychological dependence
Trade Names: Amphetamine Salt, Adderall, Adderall XR
Skin Effects: urticaria

dextroamphetamine this drug is used to treat ADHD or attention deficit hyperactivity disorder. It also is considered treatment for narcolepsy.

Side Effects: hyperactivity, insomnia, restlessness, tremors, heart palpitations, tachycardia, decreased appetite (resulting in weight loss), psychological dependence
Trade Names: Dexedrine, Dextrostat
Skin Effects: urticaria

methylphenidate used to treat ADHD or attention deficit hyperactivity disorder. It also is considered treatment for narcolepsy. It is a central nervous system stimulant.

Side Effects: changes in sleep, agitation, dizziness, painful and sour stomach, diarrhea, vomiting, changes in appetite. headaches, cough, runny nose, Uncomfortable menstruation. hyperactivity, tremor, restlessness, changes in blood pressure, changes in weight, anorexia, changes in the heart rate
Trade Name: Ritalin
Skin Effects: rash

SEDATIVES AND HYPNOTICS

Sedatives and hypnotics are most commonly used to treat sleep disorders and to act as presurgery sedatives. For your purposes, most clients using the following medications will most likely use them for the prior circumstance.

Sleep disorders are very common in the stressful times in which we live. Sleep disorders include trouble getting to sleep, trouble staying asleep, and ineffective sleep. For the millions of people who suffer from a sleep condition, medications, particularly sedatives and hypnotics, are the only resort.

Many of these medications have troubling side effects and are often habit forming.

chloral hydrate used for short term hypnotic and sedative purposes

Side Effects: extreme sedation, diarrhea, nausea, vomiting, progressively decreased tolerance, psychological and physical dependence
Trade Name: Noctec
Skin Effects: rashes

droperidol used as a tranquilizer

Side Effects: extrapyramidal reactions, hypotension, tachycardia
Trade Name: Inapsine
Skin Effects: sweating

eszopiclone long term treatment of insomnia

Side Effects: depression, hallucinations, headache, dry mouth, unpleasant taste
Trade Name: Lunesta
Skin Effects: rashes

hydroxyzine management of anxiety

Side Effects: drowsiness, dry mouth, bitter taste, constipation, nausea
Trade Name: Atarax, Hyzine-50, Vistaril
Skin Effects: flushing

ramelteon treatment of insomnia for individuals with difficult sleep onset

Side Effects: dizziness, fatigue, nausea
Trade Name: Rozerem
Skin Effects: none

zaleplon short term treatment of sleep disorders, particularly difficulty with sleep onset

Side Effects: amnesia, dizziness, drowsiness, hallucinations, headache, colitis, nausea, fatigue, vertigo, altered sense of smell and hearing, tremors
Trade Name: Sonata
Skin Effects: photosensitivity

zolpidem used to treat insomnia

Side Effects: drowsiness, dizziness, hangover, diarrhea, nausea, vomiting, physical and psychological dependence

Trade Name: Ambien, Ambien CR
Skin Effects: rashes

Conclusion

Almost 10 percent of the population in the United States suffers from one or another type of mental illness as such, the aesthetician must be alert to the medications associated with these problems. Many of the medications can cause photosensitivity, consequently education about the dangers of the sun and how their skin will be affected is critical. Furthermore the use of sun screen will be imperative in these situations. If a moisturizer with sun screen can be implemented in the home care program, compliance will be easier to achieve. There are other skin effects from these medications. Remember, that rashes can often be a result of hypersensitivity. Consequently the aesthetician should be alert to a client that begins new medication. If a rash appears, medical attention is necessary.

As we are now aware, women are at greater risk for mental illness, specifically depression. This disease is so insidious in our society it is often hard to pin point. But working with clients day to day, one becomes savvy at recognizing the symptoms. Unfortunately, there still exists a prejudice against those with mental illness, so it can be difficult to refer clients to the physician for treatment. Embarrassment, denial, the unwillingness take time out of their schedule and the symptoms of the disease contribute to a client's unwillingness to seek treatment. The aesthetician often develops a rapport with a client that is personal and intimate. This rapport often allows for an opportunity to make a referral to the physician for proper medical care.

REFERENCES

1. http://www.nlm.nih.gov
2. http://www.nimh.nih.gov
3. http://www.rxlist.com
4. http://www.drugs.com
5. Deglin, J. H., & Vallerand, A. H. (2007). *Davis's Drug Guide for Nurses.* Philadelphia, PA: F. A. Davis.
6. Michalun, N. (2001). *Milady's Skin Care and Cosmetic Ingredients Dictionary.* Clifton Park: Thomson Delmar Learning.
7. Spratto, G. R., & Woods, A. L. (2005). *2005 PDR Nurse's Drug Handbook.* Clifton Park: Thomson Delmar Learning.
8. http://www.fda.gov

CHAPTER 9

Antidiabetics

KEY TERMS

Alpha-glucosidase Inhibitors
Asthenia
Exanthema
Flatulence
Glucose
Hyperglycemia
Hypoglycemia
Incretin Mimetic Agent
Insulin
Insulin Dependent Diabetes Mellitus (IDDM)
Ketoacidosis
Lipodystrophy
Maculopapular
Meglitinides
Morbilliform
Non-insulin Dependent Diabetes Mellitus
Porphyria Cutanea Tarda
Rebound Hypoglycemia

LEARNING OBJECTIVES

After completing this chapter, you should be able to:

1. Define diabetes Type 1.
2. Define diabetes Type 2.
3. Identify the drugs that are used to treat diabetes.
4. Explain the side effects of diabetes.
5. Explain the skin effects of diabetes.

INTRODUCTION

Diabetes is a relatively common and potentially catastrophic condition that affects more than 20 million American adults or children.[1] It is a condition in which a person's blood sugar, or blood **glucose**, is too high. Glucose is a vital carbohydrate that is used by animals to supply energy to the body. While a certain amount of glucose in the blood is healthy and essential, too much can be toxic. For diabetics, a daily balancing act of calculating and responding to glucose levels is a way of life.

Our main source of glucose comes from the foods we eat; however, our liver and muscles also produce a small amount. A hormone produced in the pancreas, known as insulin, helps the cellular intake of glucose for energy. For diabetics, either they fail to produce insulin or their cells do not respond to the **insulin**. While an overabundance of glucose in the blood is the end result of diabetes, ineffectual or nonexistent insulin supplies are the root cause. For this reason, diabetics need to fortify their insulin supplies externally.

glucose
vital sugar required for normal metabolism

insulin
essential hormone needed for the normal metabolic breakdown of glucose in the body

While the exact etiology of the condition has yet to be discovered, researchers believe that genetics and environmental factors, such as obesity, contribute greatly.

There are two major types of diabetes: Type 1, or insulin dependent, diabetes and Type 2, or non-insulin dependent, diabetes. There is one other type of diabetes, gestational diabetes. Gestational diabetes occurs in pregnant woman who have high blood glucose levels. About 4 percent of women who become pregnant have gestational diabetes.[2] The cause of this

Table 9-1 Signs of Diabetes
Being very thirsty
Urinating often
Feeling very hungry or tired
Losing weight without trying
Having sores that heal slowly
Having dry, itchy skin
Losing the feeling in your feet or having tingling in your feet
Having blurry eyesight

[1]http://www.diabetes.org/diabetes-statistics.jsp
[2]http://www.diabetes.org/gestational-diabetes.jsp

phenomenon is unknown, but it is speculated that the hormones secreted by the placenta may block the insulin in the mother, causing the blood glucose levels to rise. Typically, gestational diabetes disappears after delivery, but the chances of reoccurrence are greater with future pregnancies.

TYPE 1 DIABETES

Insulin Dependent Diabetes Mellitus (IDDM)
type of diabetes in which the body cannot produce insulin or insulin is ineffective, resulting in the need for external supplies of insulin to be introduced (aka Type 1 diabetes)

hyperglycemia
increased blood sugar levels often leading to diabetic coma if unresolved

ketoacidosis
acidosis caused by abnormally high levels of ketone bodies, a compound that is a by-product of fat metabolism

hypoglycemia
abnormally low levels of glucose in the blood

Non-insulin Dependent Diabetes Mellitus
type of diabetes in which the body cannot utilize insulin, resulting in the need for monitoring or diet and exercise in addition to medication (aka Type 2 diabetes)

Type 1 diabetes, also known as **Insulin Dependent Diabetes Mellitus (IDDM),** formerly known as juvenile diabetes, is a metabolic disorder caused by a deficiency of the metabolic hormone insulin. As mentioned, this hormone is vital to the cells to convert glucose into sugar. Individuals who have IDDM can expect to have to self-administer external supplies of insulin for the rest of their lives. Because the body cannot produce its own insulin supplies, the effects of this condition are more noticeable and are often detected early in childhood. (This is the reason it was formerly called "juvenile diabetes." It is no longer referred to as such because of the increased prevalence of Type 2 diabetes in children.)

The toxic condition associated with having too much glucose in the blood is referred to as **hyperglycemia**. During a hyperglycemic episode, the individual may have shortness of breath, high glucose levels in the urine, frequent urge to urinate, and increased thirst. If left untreated, hyperglycemia could lead to a **ketoacidosis** (diabetic coma), which is a potentially serious condition. Another condition associated with Type 1 diabetes is **hypoglycemia.** This is when the body has too much insulin and not enough sugar. This is usually associated with overtreating diabetes, although one does not have to be diabetic to experience a hypoglycemic event. Symptoms of hypoglycemia include nervousness, shakiness, heart palpitations, mood swings, dilated pupils, and cold sweats. Hypoglycemia is most often treated with a controlled diet.

Having Type 1 diabetes increases your risk for many serious complications, including heart disease (cardiovascular disease), blindness (retinopathy), nerve damage (neuropathy), and kidney damage (nephropathy). In order to avoid any of these complications, routine monitoring of blood sugar levels and insulin equalization on a daily basis are necessary.

TYPE 2 DIABETES

Type 2 diabetes, or **Non-insulin Dependent Diabetes Mellitus,** is a form of diabetes in which the body is able to produce insulin, but the body has developed an insulin resistance that renders the cells unable to process the glucose for energy conversion. This condition used to be referred to as "adult onset," but a significant number of new Type 2 diabetes diagnoses are made to children and adolescents, which is due in part to the increased rates of childhood obesity.

More people have Type 2 diabetes that Type 1. It is usually managed by a combination of drugs and diet. However, like Type 1 patients, those suffering from Type 2 diabetes usually have to monitor their blood glucose levels in order to maintain stamina and to avoid long term consequences of the disease, which can be catastrophic and wide ranging. Because the body is being starved of vital energy, several consequences exist. Over time, high glucose levels will damage eyesight (leading to blindness), result in damage to the kidneys (leading to renal failure), and cause damage to nerves and heart (leading to a wide variety of consequences from heart failure to limb amputation).

While diabetes occurs in people of all ages and races, some groups have a higher risk for developing Type 2 diabetes than others. Type 2 diabetes is more common in African Americans, Latinos, Native Americans, Asian Americans/Pacific Islanders, and obese people, as well as in the aged population.

TREATMENT OF DIABETES

Treatment for diabetes is very important, regardless of which form of the disease an individual presents. Physicians will determine a treatment regime based upon several factors, including age, overall health, type of diabetes, progression of the disease, tolerance, and expectations. Both types of the disease are treated in different manners to accommodate the physical needs of the individual suffering from the condition. Regardless of which form of diabetes the individual has, diet and exercise ought to be the first line of defense.

Table 9-2 Types of Oral Medications Used to Treat Type 2 Diabetes

Type	Description
Alpha-glucosidase Inhibitors	Slow starch absorption
Biguanides	Limit the amount of sugar produced in the liver
Meglitinides	Stimulate the production of insulin
Sulfonylureas	Stimulate the production of insulin
Thiazolidinediones	Increase sensitivity to insulin

alpha-glucosidase inhibitors
group of medications used to treat diabetes by slowing the breakdown of sugars in the body

meglitinides
type of Type 2 diabetes treatment that increases insulin production in the pancreas

For individuals with Type 1 diabetes mellitus, an external supply of insulin must be administered, most often by injection. The specific form of insulin will depend on the needs of the individual and will be determined by a physician. Insulins are characterized by the time they take to work and the duration of their effectiveness.

For individuals with Type 2 diabetes, oral medications can be taken to balancetheir glucose levels when diet and exercise are no longer effective.

Alpha-glucosidase Inhibitors

acarbose used as an adjunct to diet to lower blood glucose for patients with Type 2 diabetes mellitus

Side Effects: abdominal pain, diarrhea, **flatulence**
Trade Names: Precose, Prandase
Skin Effects: hypersensitive skin, including rashes, erythema, **exanthema,** and urticaria

flatulence excessive gas

exanthema any inflamed skin eruptions

asthenia weakness or lack of strength

miglitol used to treat Type 2 diabetes in conjunction with diet and exercise

Side Effects: stomach upset, diarrhea, gas, hyperglycemia, hypoglycemia, allergy, or anaphylaxis
Trade Name: Glyset
Skin Effects: those skin reactions relating to an allergic reaction: hives, rash, itching

Biguanides

metformin hydrochloride as an adjunct to diet and exercise to reduce blood glucose

Side Effects: headache, infections, diarrhea, dyspepsia, nausea, rhinitis, flatulence, **asthenia**, indigestion, abdominal discomfort, abnormal stools, myalgia, lightheaded dyspnea, taste disorders, chest, discomfort, chills, flu syndromes, flushing palpitation
Trade Name: Glucophage
Skin Effects: nail disorders, rash, sweating

Insulins

concentrated regular insulin short acting insulin for individuals requiring >200 units per day

Side Effects: **lipodystrophy**, **rebound hypoglycemia**
Trade Names: Humulin R, Novolin R, Iletin II Regular, Velosulin BR
Skin Effects: urticaria, itching, redness, swelling (at injection site)

insulin aspart (rDNA origin) injection for the treatment of diabetes Type 1

Side Effects: allergy or anaphylaxis, hyperglycemia, hypoglycemia
Trade Name: NovoLog
Skin Effects: injection site reaction, lipodystrophy, pruritus, rash

insulin detemir long acting insulin with delayed and prolonged effects

Side Effects: lipodystrophy, rebound hypoglycemia
Trade Name: Levemir
Skin Effects: urticaria, itching, redness, swelling (at injection site)

insulin glargine long acting insulin with delayed and prolonged effects

Side Effects: lipodystrophy, rebound hypoglycemia
Trade Name: Lantus
Skin Effects: urticaria, itching, redness, swelling (at injection site)

insulin lispro rDNA origin rapid onset with shorter duration

Side Effects: lipodystrophy, rebound hypoglycemia
Trade Name: Humalog
Skin Effects: urticaria, itching, redness, swelling (at injection site)

insulin lispro/protamine insulin lispro mixture rDNA origin-mixed treatments for diabetes mellitus

Side Effects: lipodystrophy, rebound hypoglycemia
Trade Name: Humalog 75/25
Skin Effects: urticaria, itching, redness, swelling (at injection site)

insulin zinc suspension, extended (ultra-lente insulin) long acting insulin with delayed and prolonged effects
Side Effects: lipodystrophy, rebound hypoglycemia
Trade Names: Humulin U Ultralente, Novolin U, Ultralente
Skin Effects: urticaria, itching, redness, swelling (at injection site)

insulin zinc suspension (lente insulin) intermediate acting insulin treatment for diabetes mellitus

lipodystrophy
loss of fatty tissue due to defective fat metabolism

rebound hypoglycemia
phenomenon associated with decreased glucose levels following the external introduction of insulin into the body for individuals with diabetes

Side Effects: lipodystrophy, rebound hypoglycemia
Trade Names: Humulin N, NPH Iletin II, Novolin N
Skin Effects: urticaria, itching, redness, swelling (at injection site)

NPH insulin intermediate acting insulin treatment for diabetes mellitus

Side Effects: lipodystrophy, rebound hypoglycemia
Trade Names: Humulin L, Lente Iletin II
Skin Effects: urticaria, itching, redness, swelling (at injection site)

NPH/regular insulin mixture mixed treatments for diabetes mellitus

Side Effects: lipodystrophy, rebound hypoglycemia
Trade Names: Humulin 50/50, Humulin 70/30, Novolin 70/30
Skin Effects: urticaria, itching, redness, swelling (at injection site)

regular insulin short acting insulin for diabetes mellitus patients requiring >200 units per day

Side Effects: lipodystrophy, rebound hypoglycemia
Trade Names: Humulin R, Novolin R, Iletin II Regular, Velosulin BR
Skin Effects: urticaria, itching, redness, swelling (at injection site)

Meglitinides

nateglinide used to treat Type 2 diabetes in combination with diet and exercise

Side Effects: dizziness, hypoglycemia, hyperglycemia, confusion and seizures, allergy
Trade Name: Starlix
Skin Effects: rash, itching, and swelling associated with an allergic reaction

repaglinide for the treatment of Type 2 diabetes

Side Effects: hyperglycemia, hypoglycemia, diarrhea, constipation, joint pain, allergy, or anaphylaxis
Trade Name: Prandin
Skin Effects: rash or hives associated with an allergic reaction

Sulfonylureas

glimepiride used as an adjunct to diet to lower blood glucose in the treatment of Type 2 diabetes

Side Effects: dizziness, asthenia, headache, and nausea
Trade Name: Amaryl
Skin Effects: In less than 1 percent of the patients studied the following side effects were noted: pruritus, erythema, urticaria, and **morbilliform** or **maculopapular** eruptions. Also reported were **porphyria cutanea tarda**, photosensitivity, and allergic vasculitis.

morbilliform
resembling measles

maculopapular
eruptions of both macules and papules

porphyria cutanea tarda
genetic condition characterized by a disruption in normal polyphyrin metabolism

glipizide used in combination with diet and exercise to improve the levels of blood glucose, to control Type 2 diabetes

Side Effects: asthenia, headache, dizziness, nervousness, tremor, diarrhea, flatulence
Trade Name: Glucotrol XL, Glucotrol
Skin Effects: none noted

glyburide used to control blood sugar in Type 2 diabetes

Side Effects: hypoglycemia
Trade Name: DiaBeta, Glynase Pres Tab, Micronase
Skin Effects: photosensitivity and rashes

Thiazolidinediones

pioglitazone hydrochloride treats Type 2 diabetes

Side Effects: upper respiratory infections, tooth disorders, headache, sinusitis, myalgia, pharyngitis, hyperglycemia, or hypoglycemia
Trade Name: Actos
Skin Effects: none noted

rosiglitazone maleate used as a treatment for Type 2 diabetes

Side Effects: hypoglycemia, edema, changes in heartbeat
Trade Name: Avandia
Skin Effects: Urticaria

Hormone

pramlintide acetate for treatment of Type 1 and Type 2 diabetes

Side Effects: nausea, vomiting, headache, anorexia, abdominal pain, fatigue, dizziness, coughing, pharyngitis
Trade Name: Symlin
Skin Effects: none noted

incretin mimetic agent
a drug that is intended to trick the body into producing insulin as a means of treating diabetes

Incretin Mimetic Agent

exenatide for the treatment of Type 2 diabetes. Improves blood sugar. Can be used with other medications including glucophage, glimepiride, glipizide, glyburide, and others at the recommendation of the physician.

Side Effects: nausea, hypoglycemia, diarrhea, dizziness, headache, jittery feelings, upset stomach
Trade Name: Byetta
Skin Effects: welts at the injection site

Conclusion

Diabetes can be a disease that is difficult to tolerate and riddled with possible complications, but it is manageable. With the correct balance of medications, diet, and exercise, people with diabetes can live long, healthy, and prosperous lives.

While the routine of managing the condition is a delicate balance, modern medicine has enabled people with diabetes to have an even greater chance of normalcy in their daily lives. However, many of these medications have side effects that may or may not be tolerated.

For the aspiring or experienced aesthetician, this can be of consequence because many of the dermatological and aesthetic complaints of your client may be linked to the medications that the patient is taking. For continued success, during the consultative process you should compile an accurate list of medications your client uses. Cross-referencing these drugs against their side effects and possible skin effects may seem like a daunting task, but it is important to benefit the client and to ensure your success.

REFERENCES

1. http://diabetes.niddk.nih.gov/dm/pubs/type1and2/index.htm
2. http://www.emedicine.com/PED/topic581.htm
3. http://www.diabetes.org/type-1-diabetes.jsp
4. http://www.nlm.nih.gov
5. http://www.rxlist.com
6. http://www.drugs.com
7. Deglin, J. H., & Vallerand, A. H. (2007). *Davis's Drug Guide for Nurses.* Philadelphia, PA: F. A. Davis.
8. Michalun, N. (2001). *Milady's Skin Care and Cosmetic Ingredients Dictionary.* Clifton Park: Thomson Delmar Learning.

9. Roth-Skidmore, Linda. (1999). *1999 Nursing Drug Reference*. St. Louis, MO: Mosby.
10. Spratto, G. R., & Woods, A. L. (2005). *2005 PDR Nurse's Drug Handbook*. Clifton Park: Thomson Delmar Learning.
11. http://www.fda.gov
12. *Davis's Drug Guide for Nurses.*

CHAPTER 10

Antibiotics

KEY TERMS

Bactericidal Effect
Cervicitis
Diphtheria
Drug Hypersensitivities
Endocarditis
Erythrasma
Genitourinary
H. Pylori
Innocuous
Intestinal Amebiasis
Lymphocytes
Lysosomes
Meningitis
Nephrotoxicity
Pathogens
Periodontitis
Pertussis
Phototoxicity
Pyogenes Infections
Septicemia
Urethritis

LEARNING OBJECTIVES

After completing this chapter, you should be able to:

1. Explain the nature of bacterial infections.
2. Identify some of the more common bacterial infections.
3. List some of the drugs that are used to treat bacterial infections.

INTRODUCTION

Bacteria are single celled organisms that can either be **innocuous** or have far-reaching consequences for their hosts. Our bodies have evolved to include three major lines of defense to protect us from **pathogens**. The primary immune responses, the first line of defense, include **lysosomes** found in tears and saliva, enzymes in the stomach, and the acid mantel of the skin. All of these mechanisms seek to destroy or block pathogens to prevent their invasion and growth in or on the body. The next line of defense is the body's nonspecific immune responses. Immune responses use inflammation to isolate and flush out pathogens. The final line of defense is the use of **lymphocytes** to destroy specific pathogens (T-cells) and create specific immunity (B-cells). While our bodies' innate immune responses are complex and effective, many bacteria are equally cunning. Their ability to evolve quickly keeps our own mechanisms hard at work. As is often the case, an infection can outwit our own immune responses to do its damage. Until the discovery of penicillin in the 1940s, many common bacteria had devastating or dire consequences for those who contracted an infection. People lost limbs and lives due to infections that are, now, easily remedied. Because of the explosion of antibiotics in the pharmaceutical industry, this is no longer the case in the western world. However, overuse of antibiotics has caused ever-adaptable bacteria to evolve antibiotic-resistant strains that create a demand for newer and more powerful antibiotics.

MRSA, or methicillin resistant *Staphylococcus aureus,* was first discovered in the 1960s just after methicillin was introduced to the marketplace. There are five strains of MRSA in the world, and those who carry MRSA pick it up the same way as other bacteria, through physical contact, especially if the organism is on the skin. The 1990s saw a sharp rise in the number of patients infected with MRSA. MRSA is typically found in younger people and is much more likely to be the cause of a skin or soft tissue infection. Concern was raised over the past decade that MRSA was becoming antibiotic resistant, but new drugs have been developed for this very reason. Included in the list of drugs appropriate to treat MRSA infections are linezolid, quinupristin-dalfopristin, daptomycin, and others.

innocuous
without consequence

pathogens
microorganisms that produce a disease

lysosomes
a cell organelle specific to the digestive tract

lymphocytes
a blood cell

Bacteria Found in Wounds

Bacterial infections are due to the presence of microorganisms that cause damage to the tissue of its host. Most skin infections can be attributed to three pathogens: Staphylococcus, Streptococcus, and Pseudomonas.[1]

[1]http://matrix.ucdavis.edu/tumors/bacterial/bacterial.html

The extent of the damage is related to the degree of infection and particular toxin that they emit. Symptoms of a bacterial infection include inflammation, swelling, heat, and pain. People with compromised immune functions, low white blood cell counts, or malnutrition are especially vulnerable to bacterial infections.

COMMON BACTERIAL INFECTIONS

Bacterial infections usually affect a single area in the body, such as the sinuses, lungs, ears, or urinary tract. Certain bacteria produce chemicals that damage or disable parts of our bodies. In an ear infection, for example, the bacteria are in the inner ear. The body is working to fight the bacteria, but the immune system's natural processes produce inflammation. The inflammation causes pain in the inner ear. An antibiotic is prescribed to kill the bacteria. When the bacteria are eliminated, the inflammation is gone and so is the pain.

Common bacterial infections include sinusitis, strep throat, pneumonia, ear infections, and bladder infections. If untreated, a bacterial infection can spread to the bloodstream, a condition called bacteremia. This is a serious condition, one of many reasons to treat bacterial infections promptly.

HOW ANTIBIOTICS AFFECT BACTERIA

Antibiotics work to kill bacteria. Since bacteria are responsible for disease, as well as a list of unpleasant symptoms, the goal is to kill the bacteria to eliminate the disease. When our immune systems fail to take care of this matter, antibiotics are required.

In differentiating the different types of bacteria, there are two main groupings, gram positive and gram negative. Gram staining, the process used to decipher the type, is the first step to identifying the particular bacteria affecting an individual. It takes much less time than a culture and can indicate the best means of applying an appropriate treatment modality.

In reality, an antibiotic is a selective poison. It has been chosen so that it will kill the desired bacteria, but not the cells in the body. Each different type of antibiotic affects different bacteria in different ways. For example, an antibiotic might inhibit a bacterium's ability to turn glucose into energy or its ability to construct its cell wall. When this happens, the bacterium dies instead of reproducing.

ANTIBIOTIC ALLERGIES

Antibiotics are responsible for many **drug hypersensitivities** and allergies. The antibiotic category of penicillins are the most likely to cause an allergy. Often allergies to drugs will exhibit on the skin first, most likely as a rash, hives, redness, or itching. Consequently, it is important for the patient to understand that a call to the physician is important if a rash or hives show up on the skin after beginning to take an antibiotic. If an allergy is allowed to progress, it could result in swelling of the mouth and throat followed by difficulty breathing, and become a life-threatening situation. This phenomenon is called anaphylaxis.

drug hypersensitivities
abnormal reaction to a drug

bactericial effect
to destroy bacteria

nephrotoxicity
kidney toxicity

Aminoglycosides

Aminoglycosides are used for the treatment of gram-negative infections. They are also used to treat staphylococci infections when indicated. This antibiotic inhibits the synthesis of protein, causing a **bactericidal effect**. Aminoglycosides are typically effective against the following bacteria: *Pseudonomas aeruginosa, Klebsiella pneumoniae, Escherichia coli, Proteus, Serratia, Acinetobacter, Staphylococcus aureus.* These medications are given intramuscularly or intravenously. It should also be noted that cross sensitivity occurs in this category. That is to say, if an allergy exists to gentamicin, for example, it is likely that an allergy to any of the other drugs in this category will exist.

amikacin In addition to the bacteria listed, this drug is also effective against mycobacterium.

Side Effects: toxic effect on hearing, **nephrotoxicity**, possible hypersensitivity
Trade Name: Amikin
Skin Effects: none noted; skin symptoms associated with an allergic response

gentamicin

Side Effects: toxic effect on hearing, nephrotoxicity, possible hypersensitivity
Trade Name: Garamycin
Skin Effects: none noted; skin symptoms associated with an allergic response

kanamycin

Side Effects: effect on hearing, nephrotoxicity, possible hypersensitivity
Trade Name: Kantrex
Skin Effects: none noted; skin symptoms associated with an allergic response

neomycin

Side Effects: effect on hearing, nephrotoxicity, possible hypersensitivity
Trade Name: known as neomycin
Skin Effects: none noted; skin symptoms associated with an allergic response

streptomycin Like amikacin, this medication is also useful in treating *Mycobacterium.*

Side Effects: effect on hearing, nephrotoxicity, possible hypersensitivity
Trade Name: known as streptomycin
Skin Effects: none noted; skin symptoms associated with an allergic response

tobramycin

Side Effects: effect on hearing, nephrotoxicity, possible hypersensitivity
Trade Name: Nebcin
Skin Effects: none noted; skin symptoms associated with an allergic response

Carbapenems

These antibiotics are useful in treating both gram-negative and gram-positive bacterial infections. They are similar to second generation cephalosporins.

ertapenem This antibiotic is used in the treatment of intra-abdominal infections. It may also be used in the treatment of skin infections, pneumonia, complicated urinary infections, and infections associated with postpartum or gynecological matters.

Side Effects: side effects are not common
Trade Name: Invanz
Skin Effects: none noted; skin symptoms associated with an allergic response

imipenem/cilastatin This antibiotic is used for the treatment of respiratory infections, urinary infections, abdominal infections, gynecological infections, as well as infections of the skin, bones, and joints. It may also be used for **endocarditis** and bacteremia.

Side Effects: nausea, vomiting, diarrhea
Trade Name: Primaxin
Skin Effects: rash (not associated with anaphylaxis), pruritus, sweating, hives

endocarditis
inflammation of the lining of the heart

meningitis
inflammation of the membranes covering the spinal cord

septicemia
infection of the blood

meropenem This is used for the treatment of skin infections, intra-abdominal infections, and bacterial **meningitis**. This medication is given intravenously.

Side Effects: nausea, vomiting, diarrhea
Trade Name: Merrem
Skin Effects: itching

First Generation Cephalosporins

First generation cephalosporins typically have better activity against gram-positive bacteria than other antibiotics. They are frequently prescribed antibiotics, but it should be noted that up to 70 percent of the population with penicillin allergies will also have a hypersensitivity or allergy to first generation cephalosporins.

Cephalosporins are engineered to attach to the bacterial cell wall, inhibiting reproduction and causing subsequent death. They treat skin infections, pneumonia, ear infections, urinary tract infections, and bone infections. Also treated by this category is **septicemia.**

cefadroxil monohydrate This drug is used to treat individuals with infections of the skin.

Side Effects: diarrhea, nausea, vomiting; anaphylaxis is possible
Trade Names: Duricef, Ultracef
Skin Effects: rashes, urticaria, itching (not associated with an anaphylaxis)

cefazolin This antibiotic is used to treat a variety of infections. It is given intramuscularly and intravenously.

Side Effects: diarrhea, nausea, vomiting; anaphylaxis is possible
Trade Name: Ancef
Skin Effects: rashes, urticaria, itching (not associated with an anaphylaxis)

cephalexin This drug is used for the treatment of infections of the lungs, ears, bone, skin, and urinary tract.

Side Effects: diarrhea, nausea, vomiting; anaphylaxis is possible
Trade Name: Keflex
Skin Effects: rashes, urticaria, itching (not associated with an anaphylaxis)

cephradine This drug is used for the treatment of infections of the lungs, ears, bone, skin, and urinary tract.

Side Effects: diarrhea, nausea, vomiting; anaphylaxis is possible
Trade Name: Velosef
Skin Effects: rashes, urticaria, itching (not associated with anaphylaxis)

Second Generation Cephalosporins

Second generation cephalosporins treat infections similar to the first generation cephalosporins, but they are typically chosen because there is a need for broad gram-negative bacteria control. Those with serious hypersensitivity to penicillins may be allergic to this category.

cefaclor This drug is used to treat bacterial infections, especially those found in the respiratory tract: lungs and throat. It is also effective for infections found on the skin, in the urinary tract, and in the ears.

Side Effects: diarrhea, nausea, vomiting, pain at the injection site if the product is injected intramuscularly, or phlebitis if given intravenously; anaphylaxis is also possible
Trade Names: Ceclor, Ceclor CD
Skin Effects: rashes and hives (not associated with anaphylaxis)

cefotetan This drug is given intramuscularly or intravenously for the treatment of infections in the lungs, bones, skin, stomach, gynecological system, and urinary tract.

Side Effects: diarrhea, nausea, vomiting, pain at the injection site if the product is injected intramuscularly, or phlebitis if given intravenously; anaphylaxis is also possible
Trade Name: Cefotan
Skin Effects: rashes and hives (not associated with anaphylaxis)

cefoxitin This drug is given intramuscularly or intravenously for the treatment of infections in the lungs, bones, skin, stomach, gynecological system, and urinary tract.

Side Effects: diarrhea, nausea, vomiting, pain at the injection site if the product is injected intramuscularly, or phlebitis if given intravenously; anaphylaxis is also possible

Trade Name: Mefoxin
Skin Effects: rashes and hives (not associated with anaphylaxis)

cefprozil This drug is given intramuscularly or intravenously for the treatment of infections in the lungs, bones, skin, stomach, gynecological system, and urinary tract.

Side Effects: diarrhea, nausea, vomiting, pain at the injection site if the product is injected intramuscularly, or phlebitis if given intravenously; anaphylaxis is also possible
Trade Name: Cefzil
Skin Effects: rashes and hives (not associated with anaphylaxis)

cefuroxime The following infections are treated by this antibiotic: infections of the urinary tract, ears, sinus, throat, bronchi, as well as Lyme disease and gonorrhea.

Side Effects: diarrhea, nausea, vomiting, pain at the injection site if the product is injected intramuscularly, or phlebitis if given intravenously; anaphylaxis is also possible
Trade Names: Ceftin, Zinacef
Skin Effects: rashes and hives (not associated with anaphylaxis)

loracarbef This antibiotic is used to treat infections of the lungs, ears, nose, throat, skin, and urinary tract.

Side Effects: diarrhea, nausea, vomiting, pain at the injection site if the product is injected intramuscularly, or phlebitis if given intravenously; anaphylaxis is also possible
Trade Name: Lorabid
Skin Effects: rashes and hives (not associated with anaphylaxis)

Third Generation Cephalosporins

The third generation of cephalosporins is similar to the first and second generations but has the best control over gram-negative bacteria.

cefdinir This drug treats infections in the lungs and bronchi, infections of the skin, and septicemia, as well as ear, bone, urinary, and gynecological infections.

Side Effects: diarrhea, nausea, vomiting, pain at the injection site, or phlebitis at the intravenous site
Trade Name: Omnicef
Skin Effects: rash and hives (not associated with anaphylaxis)

cefditoren This drug treats infections in the lungs and bronchi, infections of the skin, and septicemia, as well as ear, bone, urinary, and gynecological infections. This medication is especially useful in recurrent cases of bronchitis.

Side Effects: diarrhea, nausea, vomiting, pain at the injection site, or phlebitis at the intravenous site
Trade Name: Spectracef
Skin Effects: rash and hives (not associated with anaphylaxis)

cefepime This drug treats infections in the lungs and bronchi, infections of the skin, and septicemia, as well as ear, bone, urinary, and gynecological infections. The medication can be administered orally, injected intramuscularly, and given intravenously.

Side Effects: diarrhea, nausea, vomiting, pain at the injection site, or phlebitis at the intravenous site
Trade Name: Maxipime
Skin Effects: rash and hives (not associated with anaphylaxis)

cefoperazone This drug treats infections in the lungs and bronchi, infections of the skin, and septicemia, as well as ear, bone, urinary, and gynecological infections. The medication can be administered orally, injected intramuscularly, and given intravenously.

Side Effects: diarrhea, nausea, vomiting, pain at the injection site, or phlebitis at the intravenous site
Trade Name: Cefobid
Skin Effects: rash and hives (not associated with anaphylaxis)

cefotaxime This drug treats infections in the lungs and bronchi, infections of the skin, and septicemia, as well as ear, bone, urinary, and gynecological infections. This medication can also treat meningitis and Lyme disease. The medication can be administered orally, injected intramuscularly, and given intravenously.

Side Effects: diarrhea, nausea, vomiting, pain at the injection site, or phlebitis at the intravenous site
Trade Name: Claforan
Skin Effects: rash and hives (not associated with anaphylaxis)

cefpodoxime This drug treats infections in the lungs and bronchi, infections of the skin, and septicemia, as well as ear, bone, urinary, and gynecological infections. Meningitis can also be treated with this medication. The medication can be administered orally, injected intramuscularly, and given intravenously.

Side Effects: diarrhea, nausea, vomiting, pain at the injection site, or phlebitis at the intravenous site

Trade Name: Vantin
Skin Effects: rash and hives (not associated with anaphylaxis)

ceftazidime This drug treats infections in the lungs and bronchi, infections of the skin, and septicemia, as well as ear, bone, urinary, and gynecological infections. The medication can be administered orally, injected intramuscularly, and given intravenously.

Side Effects: diarrhea, nausea, vomiting, pain at the injection site, or phlebitis at the intravenous site
Trade Names: Fortaz, Tazicef
Skin Effects: rash and hives (not associated with anaphylaxis)

ceftibuten This drug treats infections in the lungs and bronchi, infections of the skin, and septicemia, as well as ear, bone, urinary, and gynecological infections.

Side Effects: diarrhea, nausea, vomiting, pain at the injection site, or phlebitis at the intravenous site
Trade Name: Cedax
Skin Effects: rash and hives (not associated with anaphylaxis)

cefditoren This drug treats infections in the lungs and bronchi, infections of the skin, and septicemia, as well as ear, bone, urinary, and gynecological infections. The medication can be administered orally, injected intramuscularly, and given intravenously.

Side Effects: diarrhea, nausea, vomiting, pain at the injection site, or phlebitis at the intravenous site
Trade Name: Spectracef
Skin Effects: rash and hives (not associated with anaphylaxis)

ceftriaxone This drug treats infections in the lungs and bronchi, infections of the skin, and septicemia, as well as ear, bone, urinary, and gynecological infections. This medication can also treat meningitis and Lyme disease. The medication can be administered orally, injected intramuscularly, and given intravenously.

Side Effects: diarrhea, nausea, vomiting, pain at the injection site, or phlebitis at the intravenous site
Trade Name: Rocephin
Skin Effects: rash and hives (not associated with anaphylaxis)

Extended Spectrum Penicillins

This group of penicillins typically treats more serious infections. The focus of this category of drugs is gram-negative bacteria.

piperacillin This medication treats more serious infections of the skin, bone, and lungs, as well as septicemia, gynecological infections, intra-abdominal infections, and urinary tract infections. This medication is given intravenously and intramuscularly.

Side Effects: hypokalemia, pain at the injection sites, or phlebitis at intravenous site; anaphylaxis is possible
Trade Name: Pipracil
Skin Effects: rashes, especially in patients with cystic fibrosis, hives

piperacillin/tazobactam This medication is used for patients with appendicitis, skin infections, and gynecological infections.

Side Effects: hypokalemia, pain at the injection sites, or phlebitis at intravenous site; anaphylaxis is possible
Trade Name: Zosyn
Skin Effects: rashes, especially in patients with cystic fibrosis, hives

ticarcillin This medication treats skin infections, bone infections, respiratory tract infections, gynecological infections, urinary tract infections, and septicemia. This medication is given intramuscularly and intravenously.

Side Effects: diarrhea, hypokalemia, phlebitis at the intravenous site; anaphylaxis is possible
Trade Name: Ticar
Skin Effects: rashes and hives (not related to anaphylaxis)

ticarcillin/clavulanate This medication treats skin infections, bone infections, respiratory tract infections, gynecological infections, urinary tract infections, and septicemia.

Side Effects: diarrhea, hypokalemia, phlebitis at the intravenous site; anaphylaxis is possible
Trade Name: Timentin
Skin Effects: rashes and hives (not related to anaphylaxis)

Fluoroquinolones

Quinolones are useful in a broad category of bacteria. They also work well in combination with aminoglycosides, rifampin, and carbapenems.

ciprofloxacin This product is used to treat infections of the lung, bones, skin, prostate, sinus, and urinary tracts, as well as bronchitis, prostate gonorrhea, diarrhea (bacterial), typhoid fever, and anthrax.

Side Effects: dizziness, drowsiness, headache, insomnia, abdominal pain, diarrhea, nausea; anaphylaxis is possible.

Trade Name: Cipro, Cipro XR
Skin Effects: photosensitivity, rash, **phototoxicity**

phototoxicity
a harmful reaction from the sun

gatifloxacin This antibiotic is commonly used to treat infections of the skin, lungs, respiratory tract, and urinary tract, as well as sexually transmitted diseases.

Side Effects: dizziness, drowsiness, headache, insomnia, abdominal pain, diarrhea, nausea; anaphylaxis is possible
Trade Name: Tequin
Skin Effects: photosensitivity, rash, phototoxicity

gemofloxacin This product is used to treat infections of the lung, bones, skin, prostate, sinus, and urinary tracts, as well as bronchitis, gonorrhea, diarrhea (bacterial), typhoid fever, and anthrax.

Side Effects: dizziness, drowsiness, headache, insomnia, abdominal pain, diarrhea, nausea; anaphylaxis is possible
Trade Name: Factive
Skin Effects: photosensitivity, rash, phototoxicity

levofloxacin This is an antibiotic used to treat infections of the lungs, sinuses, kidneys, prostate, urinary tract, and skin.

Side Effects: dizziness, drowsiness, headache, insomnia, abdominal pain, diarrhea, nausea; anaphylaxis is possible
Trade Name: Levaquin
Skin Effects: photosensitivity, rash, phototoxicity

lomefloxacin This is an antibiotic used to treat infections of the lungs, sinuses, kidneys, urinary tract, and skin.

Side Effects: dizziness, drowsiness, headache, insomnia, abdominal pain, diarrhea, nausea; anaphylaxis is possible
Trade Name: Maxaquin
Skin Effects: photosensitivity, rash, phototoxicity

moxifloxacin This is an antibiotic used to treat infections of the lungs, sinuses, kidneys, urinary tract, and skin.

Side Effects: dizziness, drowsiness, headache, insomnia, abdominal pain, diarrhea, nausea; anaphylaxis is possible
Trade Name: Avelox
Skin Effects: photosensitivity, rash, phototoxicity

norfloxacin This is an antibiotic used to treat infections of the kidneys, urinary tract, and skin.

Side Effects: dizziness, drowsiness, headache, insomnia, abdominal pain, diarrhea, nausea; anaphylaxis is possible
Trade Name: Noroxin
Skin Effects: photosensitivity, rash, phototoxicity

ofloxacin This antibiotic is used to treat infections of the lungs, prostate, skin, and urinary tract, as well as sexually transmitted diseases.

Side Effects: dizziness, drowsiness, headache, insomnia, abdominal pain, diarrhea, nausea; anaphylaxis is possible
Trade Name: Floxin
Skin Effects: photosensitivity, rash, phototoxicity

Macrolides

The most commonly prescribed macrolides are erythromycin, azithromycin, and clarithromycin. These antibiotics interfere with protein synthesis in the bacterial cell.

urethritis
inflammation of the urethra

cervicitis
inflammation of the cervix

H. pylori
Helicobacter Pylori bacteria involved in digestive illness

pertussis
whooping cough

diphtheria
infection of the mucous membranes

erythrasma
infectious skin eruptions under the arm and in the groin

intestinal amebiasis
infection of the intestine caused by *Entamoeba histolytica*

azithromycin This medication is used in the treatment of respiratory infections, ear infections, skin infections, **urethritis**, **cervicitis,** and sexually transmitted diseases, such as gonorrhea. It also treats cystic fibrosis and endocarditis.

Side Effects: abdominal pain, diarrhea, nausea
Trade Names: Zithromax, Z-pak
Skin Effects: photosensitivity, Stevens-Johnson syndrome, rashes

clarithromycin This medication is used to treat infections in the lungs, bronchi, ears, sinuses, skin, and throat. It is also used to treat *Mycobacterium avium* complex in those individuals with HIV and ***H. pylori***.

Side Effects: side effects are not common to this medication
Trade Name: Biaxin
Skin Effects: skin effects are not common to this medication

erythromycin base This medication is used to treat the following: infections of the skin, urinary tract, lungs, intestines, and ears, as well as sexually transmitted diseases, rheumatic fever, **pertussis, diphtheria, erythrasma**, **intestinal amebiasis**, pelvic inflammatory disease, and Legionnaires' disease.

Side Effects: nausea, vomiting, and phlebitis at the intravenous site, if given intravenously
Trade Names: E-Base, E-Mycin, Eryc, Ery-Tab, PCE
Skin Effects: skin effects are not common to this medication

erythromycin estolate This medication is used to treat the following: infections of the skin, urinary tract, lungs, intestines, and ears, as well as sexually transmitted diseases, rheumatic fever, pertussis, diphtheria, erythrasma, intestinal amebiasis, pelvic inflammatory disease, and Legionnaires' disease

Side Effects: nausea, vomiting, and phlebitis at the intravenous site, if given intravenously
Trade Name: Ilosone
Skin Effects: skin effects are not common to this medication

erythromycin ethylsuccinate This medication is used to treat the following: infections of the skin, urinary tract, lungs, intestines, and ears, as well as sexually transmitted diseases, rheumatic fever, pertussis, diphtheria, erythrasma, intestinal amebiasis, pelvic inflammatory disease, and Legionnaires' disease.

Side Effects: nausea, vomiting and phlebitis at the intravenous site, if given intravenously
Trade Names: E.E.S., EryPed
Skin Effects: skin effects are not common to this medication

erythromycin gluceptate This medication is used to treat the following: infections of the skin, urinary tract, lungs, intestines, and ears, as well as sexually transmitted diseases, rheumatic fever, pertussis, diphtheria, erythrasma, intestinal amebiasis, pelvic inflammatory disease, and Legionnaires' disease.

Side Effects: nausea, vomiting, and phlebitis at the intravenous site, if given intravenously
Trade Name: known as erythromycin gluceptate
Skin Effects: skin effects are not common to this medication

erythromycin lactobionate This medication is used to treat the following: infections of the skin, urinary tract, lungs, intestines, and ears, as well as sexually transmitted diseases, rheumatic fever, pertussis, diphtheria, erythrasma, intestinal amebiasis, pelvic inflammatory disease, and Legionnaires' disease.

Side Effects: nausea, vomiting, and phlebitis at the intravenous site, if given intravenously
Trade Name: Erythrocin
Skin Effects: skin effects are not common to this medication

erythromycin stearate This medication is used to treat the following: infections of the skin, urinary tract, lungs, intestines, and ears, as well assexually transmitted diseases, rheumatic fever, pertussis, diphtheria, erythrasma, intestinal amebiasis, pelvic inflammatory disease, and Legionnaires' disease.

Side Effects: nausea, vomiting, and phlebitis at the intravenous site, if given intravenously
Trade Name: Erythrocin
Skin Effects: skin effects are not common to this medication

erythromycin topicals This medication is used for the treatment of acne.

Side Effects: side effects only localized
Trade Names: A/T/S, E/Gel, Emgel, Erycette, Erygel, EryMax, Theramycin Z, T-Stat
Skin Effects: irritation and redness at the site

Penicilllins

Penicillin is sometimes abbreviated PCN by medical personnel. This medication is very active on gram-positive bacteria. Developed during WWII, penicillin saved many lives that would have previously succumbed to infection.

genitourinary
to describe the organs of the urinary tract and the reproductive organs

amoxicillin This medication is used for the treatment of skin infections, ear infections, respiratory infections, sinusitis, **genitourinary** infections, and management of *H. Pylori.*

Side Effects: diarrhea, possible anaphylaxis
Trade Names: Amoxil, Trimox, Wymox
Skin Effects: rashes and hives

amoxicillin/clavulanate This medication is used for the treatment of skin infections, ear infections, sinusitis, respiratory infections, and genitourinary tract infections.

Side Effects: diarrhea, possible anaphylaxis
Trade Names: Augmentin, Augmentin ES, Augmentin XR
Skin Effects: rashes and hives

ampicillin This medication is used for the treatment of skin infections, ear infections, sinusitis, respiratory infections, genitourinary tract infections, meningitis, and septicemia.

Side Effects: diarrhea, possible anaphylaxis
Trade Name: Omnipen
Skin Effects: rashes and hives

ampicillin/sulbactam This medication is used for the treatment of skin infections, ear infections, sinusitis, respiratory infections, genitourinary tract infections, meningitis, and septicemia.

Side Effects: diarrhea, nausea, vomiting
Trade Name: Unasyn
Skin Effects: rashes and hives

benzathine penicillin G This penicillin product treats a wide variety of infectious situations, including pneumonia, streptococcal infections, syphilis, gonorrhea, and Lyme disease.

Side Effects: diarrhea, epigastric distress, nausea, vomiting, pain at the site of an intramuscular injection, phlebitis at the site of an intravenous injection
Trade Names: Bilcillin L-A, Permapen
Skin Effects: rashes and hives

cloxacillin This medication is used to treat sinusitis, skin infections, and respiratory tract infections.

Side Effects: diarrhea, nausea; anaphylaxis is possible
Trade Name: Cloxapen
Skin Effects: rash and hives

dicloxacillin This medication is used to treat sinusitis, skin infections, and respiratory tract infections.

Side Effects: diarrhea, nausea; anaphylaxis is possible
Trade Names: Dycill, Dynapen
Skin Effects: rash and hives

nafcillin This medication is used to treat sinusitis, skin infections, respiratory tract infections, bone infections, urinary tract infections, endocarditis, septicemia, and meningitis.

Side Effects: diarrhea, nausea; anaphylaxis is possible
Trade Name: Unipen
Skin Effects: rash and hives

oxacillin This medication is used to treat sinusitis, skin infections, respiratory tract infections, bone infections, urinary tract infections, endocarditis, septicemia, and meningitis.

Side Effects: diarrhea, nausea; anaphylaxis is possible
Trade Name: Bactocill
Skin Effects: rash and hives

penicillin V This penicillin product treats a wide variety of infectious situations, including pneumonia, streptococcal infections, syphilis, gonorrhea, and Lyme disease.

Side Effects: diarrhea, epigastric distress, nausea, vomiting, pain at the site of an intramuscular injection, phlebitis at the site of an intravenous injection
Trade Names: Pen-VeeK, Veetids
Skin Effects: rashes and hives

penicillin G This penicillin product treats a wide variety of infectious situations, including pneumonia, streptococcal infections, syphilis, gonorrhea, and Lyme disease.

Side Effects: diarrhea, epigastric distress, nausea, vomiting, pain at the site of an intramuscular injection, phlebitis at the site of an intravenous injection
Trade Name: Pfizerpen
Skin Effects: rashes and hives

procaine penicillin G This penicillin product treats a wide variety of infectious situations, including pneumonia, streptococcal infections, syphilis, gonorrhea, and Lyme disease.

Side Effects: diarrhea, epigastric distress, nausea, vomiting, pain at the site of an intramuscular injection, phlebitis at the site of an intravenous injection
Trade Name: Wycillin
Skin Effects: rashes and hives

Sulfonamides

Sulfonamides or sulfa antibiotics have long played a role in the management of infections typically in the urinary tract. But over the years organisms have developed a resistance to this antibiotic. Recently MRSA is treated with sulfonamides in combination with other medications.

trimethoprim/sulfamethoxazole This is typically an injectable or intravenous antibiotic used to treat bacterial infections of the lungs, ears, urinary tract, and bowel.

Side Effects: nausea, vomiting, phlebitis at the intravenous site
Trade Names: Bactrim DS, Septra, Septra DS
Skin Effects: toxic epidermal necrolysis, rashes, photosensitivity, erythema multiform

Tetracyclines

Tetracyclines work by blocking protein synthesis. Because this medication needs an acidic environment for absorption, it is important to review the diet of the patient prior to taking this medication: no milk, antacids, or other substances that would change the acid base of the stomach. Tetracyclines deposit in bones and teeth of growing children and therefore should not be prescribed for children under seven.

doxycycline This medication is used to treat unusual infections. It covers organisms that are also managed by penicillin, giving those who are allergic to penicillin another option. Common uses are to treat acne, **periodontitis**, anthrax, gonorrhea, and syphilis.

periodontitis
inflammation of the dental periosteum

Side Effects: dizziness, diarrhea, nausea, vomiting
Trade Names: Doryx, Monodox, Vibramycin, Vibra Tabs
Skin Effects: photosensitivity, rashes

minocycline This is an antibiotic used to treat infections such as acne or skin infections. It is also used for infections of the lungs and urinary systems, as well as infections associated with the central nervous system.

Side Effects: vestibular reactions, dizziness, diarrhea, nausea, vomiting
Trade Names: Dynacin, Minocin
Skin Effects: photosensitivity, rashes, pigmentation of the skin

tetracycline This medication is used to treat bacterial infection; it is directed usually at the treatment of acne.

Side Effects: dizziness, diarrhea, nausea, vomiting
Trade Names: Achromycin, Sumycin
Skin Effects: photosensitivity, rashes

Miscellaneous

These miscellaneous antibiotics do not fit any category identified above.

clindamycin This antibiotic is used to treat infections of the respiratory tract, skin, pelvis, vagina, and abdomen.

Side Effects: vomiting and nausea, flatulence, diarrhea
Trade Names: Cleocin T, Cleocin
Skin Effects: rash

drotrecogin This medication is used in the treatment of sepsis.

Side Effects: none noted
Trade Name: Xigris
Skin Effects: none noted

pyogenes infections
producing pus

linezolid This medication is used to treat uncomplicated skin infections, *Staphylococcus aureus*, *Streptococcus pneumonieae*, and *Streptococcus* ***pyogenes*** **infections.**

Side Effects: side effects are not common
Trade Name: Zyvox
Skin Effects: side effects are not common

metronidazole This medication is an antibiotic used to treat infections.

Side Effects: diarrhea, vertigo, headache, stomach pain, vomiting, anorexia
Trade Names: Flagyl, Metrocream, Metrogel, Metrogel-Vaginal, MetroLotion
Skin Effects: rash and hives with topical use, burning, mild dryness, skin irritation, transient redness

mupirocin This medication is used in the treatment of impetigo, infected skin injuries, and nasal colonization of methicillin resistant *S. aureus.*

Side Effects: uncommon
Trade Names: Bactroban, Bactroban Nasal
Skin Effects: with topical use only: burning, stinging, itching, pain

nitrofurantoin This antibiotic is used for the treatment of urinary tract infection.

Side Effects: anorexia, nausea, vomiting and hypersensitivity
Trade Names: Furadantin, Macrobid, Macrodantin
Skin Effects: photosensitivity

quinupristin/dalfopristin This medication is used in life-threatening situations when infections are vancomycin-resistant *Enterococcus faecium* and is also used for complicated skin infections.

Side Effects: uncommon swelling and inflammation at the intravenous site
Trade Name: Synercid
Skin Effects: rash and itching

rifaximin This medication is used for the treatment of traveler's diarrhea.

Side Effects: dizziness
Trade Name: Xifaxan
Skin Effects: none noted

telithromycin This medication is used to treat acute bronchitis and sinusitis.

Side Effects: diarrhea
Trade Name: Ketek
Skin Effects: none noted

trimethoprim This medication is used for the treatment of urinary tract infections.

Side Effects: changes in taste, stomachaches, swollen tongue, nausea, vomiting
Trade Name: Trimpex
Skin Effects: rash and itching

vancomycin This medication is used to treat staphylococcal infections of the heart, bones, muscles, lungs, and soft tissue, as well as in the treatment of meningitis. It is commonly used when patients are allergic to penicillin.

Side Effects: nephrotoxicity, phlebitis at the intravenous site
Trade Name: Vancocin
Skin Effects: rashes

Conclusion

Antibiotics are some of the most commonly used prescription drugs in the United States. For the aspiring aesthetician, this can be particularly relevant to the procedures that are performed in the spa environment. In the spa an aesthetician might come in contact with patients who have an infection. Infections could be as minor as acne or as significant as MRSA. The aesthetician should consider the antibiotic the patient is taking and the reason for the prescription. Because many of the skin complaints could actually be side effects of antibiotics that the patient is taking, it is vital to be knowledgeable about the patient's conditions and medications. This can be best accomplished during the consultative process. Taking a few moments to cross-reference these medications with the possible skin effects will help you to help your clients.

REFERENCES

1. Lesher, J., & Woody, C. M. (2003). Antimicrobial Drugs. In J. Bolognia, J. Jorizzo, & R. Rapini (Eds.), *Dermatology* (pp. 2007–2031). Philadelphia, PA: Mosby.

2. Deglin, J. H., & Vallerand, A. H. (2007). *Davis's Drug Guide for Nurses.* Philadelphia, PA: F. A. Davis.
3. http://www.nlm.nih.gov
4. http://www.rxlist.com
5. http://www.drugs.com
6. Michalun, N. (2001). *Milady's Skin Care and Cosmetic Ingredients Dictionary.* Clifton Park: Thomson Delmar Learning.
7. Spratto, G. R., & Woods, A. L. (2005). 2005 *PDR Nurse's Drug Handbook.* Clifton Park: Thomson Delmar Learning.
8. http://www.fda.gov

Antivirals and Antiretrovirals

CHAPTER 11

Antivirals and Antiretrovirals

KEY TERMS

Alopecia
Arthralgia
Cytomegalovirus Retinitis
Eczematoid Dermatitis
Granulocytopenia
Hantavirus
Hemolytic Anemia
Hyperglycemia
Hyperlipidemia
Hypocalcemia
Hypokalemia
Hypomagnesemia
Mottling
Myalgia
Neuropathy
Neutropenia
Proteinura
Renal Failure
Thrombocytopenia
Unicellular
Vitreous Hemorrhage

LEARNING OBJECTIVES

After completing this chapter, you should be able to:

1. Explain the nature of viral infections.
2. Identify some of the more common cutaneous viral infections.
3. List some of the drugs that are used to treat viral infections.

INTRODUCTION

unicellular
pertaining to only one cell

Hantavirus
virus that is transmitted to humans through rodent feces with potentially fatal consequences

Viruses are **unicellular** entities that straddle the fence between living and nonliving. They exist everywhere there are cells to infect. They are in the air, in soil, and in water. They exist for one purpose and one purpose only: to reproduce. There are thousands of different types of viruses. Some infect plants, some infect animals, and some even infect bacteria. They have a variety of shapes and sizes, but they are all microscopic.

Viruses are basically a microscopic bundle of genetic material (either DNA or RNA) housed within an envelope. They float around, in an inert state, waiting to attach to a suitable host cell that they then infect and commandeer. Once they have infected a host cell, they use the operations of the cell to reproduce. However, viruses are rather picky about what type of cells they infect. Viruses that infect plants are capable of infecting animals, and vice versa. In addition, viruses that infect one species can easily move to a closely related species. Furthermore, viruses behave differently in different species. An example of this would be the **Hantavirus**. Hantavirus infects rodents with no apparent detriment. Once it infects humans, however, the results are often fatal.

The body has means to protect itself from viruses. One such means is the skin itself. The skin acts as a barrier to hold what is needed in and keep what is not needed out. However, being the opportunistic entities that they are, viruses are adept at finding alternative entries to the body. Once it has found means to enter the body, the virus is fought by the body's internal mechanisms. Those mechanisms are known as our immunities. White blood cells begin to fight the virus. If the virus does not survive this battle, the white blood cells respond by remembering the virus, and the means to defeat it, rendering an individual immune to further infection.

Vaccination is another means of combating viruses. By introducing a small, easily combated dose of the virus into the body, it develops the immunity before a full-blown attack.

COMMON VIRAL INFECTIONS

In humans, the viruses have a wide variety of physical expressions. Since viruses usually infect only one type of cell, different viruses will have different expressions. For instance, the virus that causes the common cold infects only respiratory cells, or the virus that causes AIDS affects only immune system cells.

The types of viruses that cause the more common skin diseases are the herpes simplex virus and the papilloma virus. Together, these viruses are responsible for cold sores (HSV-1), genital herpes (HSV-2), and warts (HPV). Viruses that are responsible for respiratory distress are upper respiratory. They include the common cold, influenza, and sinusitis. A few viruses infect the nervous system, but they are rare. They include encephalitis and West Nile Virus.

Treating viruses poses a unique challenge. Unlike bacterial infections, in which antibiotics can target the infecting agent, viruses are more difficult to treat since they are in a constant state of genetic flux. Drugs that are used to treat viruses are called antivirals. Since viruses reside in commandeered cells, and replicate by means of those cells, antiviral drugs target the DNA of infected cells to hinder replication. As a consequence, antiviral drugs are much more expensive to develop. Furthermore, viruses can develop a resistance to antiviral drugs, requiring a constant influx of new antiviral drugs.

Human immunodeficiency virus (HIV) is a virus that disables specific immune cell functioning. When HIV is contracted, it attacks the cells that provide immunity for the body, causing a gradual deterioration of immune defenses. The cells that are typically attacked by the virus are the T-cells and CD2+ cells. Eventually the body's immunity becomes seriously compromised, and at that point the disease is called acquired immunodeficiency syndrome (AIDS). HIV and AIDS are treated with antiretrovirals, which have been developed specifically to fight the virus.

Antivirals

Antivirals are specific in their treatment. There are five target viral situations that are controlled by the drugs in this category: herpes virus infections, chicken pox, influenza, **cytomegalovirus retinitis,** and ophthalmic viral infections.

cytomegalovirus retinitis
type of herpes virus that can have potentially catastrophic effects on pregnancy

acyclovir This drug is used to treat the pain and improve the healing of cold sores. The application is also useful for chicken pox and herpes zoster. This drug is also used in the treatment of individuals with genital herpes.

Side Effects: stomach upset, nausea, vomiting, diarrhea, vertigo, headache, pain, and phlebitis
Trade Name: Zovarix
Skin Effects: acne, hives, rashes, sweating, Stevens-Johnson syndrome, hair loss

amantadine hydrochloride This drug is used as a prophylaxis and management of influenza A virus.

Side Effects: nausea, vertigo, jerky muscle movements, and changes in sleep

Trade Name: Symmetrel
Skin Effects: **mottling**, rashes are possible. Rarely **eczematoid dermatitis** will occur.

cidofovir This is an antiviral. It is usually used to help manage cytomegalovirus of the eyes in patients with AIDS.

Side Effects: headache, weakness and loss of strength, difficulty breathing, stomachache, nausea, vomiting, fever, chills, infections, **neutropenia,** and **proteinura**
Trade Name: Vistide
Skin Effects: **alopecia**, rash

docosanol This antiviral is used to treat oral and facial herpes. It is applied topically.

Side Effects: side effects are on the skin only because this is topical
Trade Name: Abreva
Skin Effects: acne, itching, rash

entecavir This medication is used in the treatment of chronic hepatitis B infections.

Side Effects: dizziness, fatigue, headache, upset stomach, nausea
Trade Name: Baraclude
Skin Effects: none noted

famciclovir This medication is used to treat shingles and genital herpes.

Side Effects: stomach upset, nausea, vomiting, diarrhea, headache, dizziness, fatigue
Trade Name: Famvir
Skin Effects: none noted

foscarnet

Side Effects: headache, diarrhea, nausea, vomiting, **renal failure**, **hypocalcemia**, **hypokalemia**, **hypomagnesemia**, anemia, **arthralgia**, **myalgia**, fever
Trade Name: Foscavir
Skin Effects: increased sweating, pruritus, rash, skin ulceration

ganciclovir This medication is used to treat cytomegalovirus retinitis.

Side Effects: decreased vision, **vitreous hemorrhage**, neutropenia, **thrombocytopenia**
Trade Names: Cytovene, Vitrasert
Skin Effects: dry, itchy skin, alopecia, photosensitivity

mottling
skin condition characterized by discoloration of the skin

eczematoid dermatitis
itchiness and redness of the skin resulting from eczema

neutropenia
abnormally low levels of neutrophil cells in the body

proteinura
high levels of protein in the urine

alopecia
hair loss

renal failure
inability of the kidneys to function normally

hypocalcemia
abnormally low levels of calcium in the blood

hypokalemia
abnormally low levels of potassium in the blood

hypomagnesemia
abnormally low levels of magnesium in the blood accompanied by muscle irritability

arthralgia
joint pain

myalgia
muscle pain

vitreous hemorrhage
bleeding in the eye

thrombocytopenia
abnormal decrease in blood platelet levels

lamivudine This medication is used in the treatment of HIV and hepatitis B.

Side Effects: fatigue, headache, trouble sleeping, lethargy, cough, anorexia, diarrhea, nausea, vomiting, muscle pain, bone pain, **neuropathy**
Trade Names: Epivir, Epivir HBV, 3TC
Skin Effects: alopecia, erythema multiforme, rashes, hives

neuropathy
disease of the brain or brain function

hemolytic anemia
low iron levels resulting from the destruction of red blood cells

oseltamivir This medication is used for the treatment of acute influenza.

Side Effects: trouble sleeping, dizziness, bronchitis, nausea, vomiting
Trade Name: Tamiflu
Skin Effects: none noted

penciclovir This medication is used topically for cold sores and herpes simplex virus.

Side Effects: headache
Trade Name: Denavir
Skin Effects: irritation at the site of application

ribavirin This medication is used to manage hepatitis C, and it is usually used in conjunction with interferon.

Side Effects: **hemolytic anemia,** shortness of breath, anorexia
Trade Names: Rebetol, Copegus, Virazole
Skin Effects: rash, itching

valacyclovir This medication is used to treat herpes zoster, also known as shingles, and herpes simplex.

Side Effects: headache, nausea, diarrhea, constipation, dizziness, weakness, anorexia, stomach pain
Trade Name: Valtrex
Skin Effects: none noted

valganciclovir hydrochloride This medication is used to treat viral infections, specifically cytomegalovirus retinitis.

Side Effects: headache, insomnia, stomach pain, nausea, vomiting, diarrhea, anemia, and fever
Trade Name: Valcyte
Skin Effects: hives

vidarabine This medication is used to treat viral infections of the eye.

Side Effects: commonly the eyes will tear and overflow; also swelling, itching, redness, burning, pain, and sensitivity to light

Trade Name: Vira-A
Skin Effects: none noted

zanamivir This medication is used to manage influenza.

Side Effects: bronchospasm
Trade Name: Relenza
Skin Effects: none noted

ANTIRETROVIRALS

There are four categories of antiretrovirals: nonnucleoside reverse transcriptase inhibitors, nucleoside reverse transcriptase inhibitors, protease inhibitors, and fusion inhibitors. Each drug functions differently but helps to treat HIV and AIDS. Both nonnucleoside reverse transcriptase inhibitors and nucleoside reverse transcriptase inhibitors work by prohibiting the HIV enzyme from converting HIV RNA to HIV DNA. Protease inhibitors work in a completely different way by interfering with the protease enzyme that HIV uses to produce infectious viral particles. Finally, fusion inhibitors work to interfere with the virus's ability to fuse cellular membrane. This action blocks the entry to the cell's host. Knowing these different drug functions, it is easy to see why a patient might be on a "cocktail" of several drugs to manage his or her disease.

Nonnucleoside Reverse Transcriptase Inhibitors

These drugs have a very specific function: to interfere with the processes of RNA conversion to DNA.

delavirdine mesylate This medication is used to manage HIV-1 infection. It is typically used with other antiviral drugs.

Side Effects: headache, fatigue, diarrhea
Trade Name: Rescriptor
Skin Effects: rash

efavirenz This medication is used in concert with other medications in the treatment of HIV.

Side Effects: nausea
Trade Name: Sustiva
Skin Effects: rash

nevirapine This medication is used for the treatment of HIV.

Side Effects: headache, elevated liver enzymes, nausea, fever
Trade Name: Viramune
Skin Effects: rash

Nucleoside Reverse Transcriptase Inhibitors

These medications are slightly different from the nonnucleoside reverse transcriptase inhibitors. This medication's job is to prevent the completion of the DNA chain.

abacavir This drug is use for the treatment of HIV-1 infections. It keeps the virus from reproducing or converting to AIDS.

Side Effects: diarrhea, nausea, vomiting, anorexia, headache, trouble sleeping
Trade Name: Ziagen
Skin Effects: rash

didanosine This medication is used to treat HIV infected individuals who may or may not have converted to AIDS. It is a transcriptase inhibitor.

Side Effects: headache, rhinitis, cough, anorexia, diarrhea, liver function abnormalities, nausea, vomiting, **granulocytopenia**, neuropathy in the arms and legs, chills, and fever
Trade Names: ddl, dideoxyinosine, Videx, Videx EC
Skin Effects: alopecia, ecchymoses, rash

granulocytopenia abnormally low levels of granulocytes in the blood

emtricitabine This medication is used in the treatment of HIV.

Side Effects: dizziness, headache, trouble sleeping, weakness, abdominal pain, diarrhea, nausea, cough
Trade Name: Emtriva
Skin Effects: rash, skin discoloration

stavudine This medication is used for the treatment of HIV.

Side Effects: headache, trouble sleeping, weakness, neuropathy of the arms and legs
Trade Names: Zerit, Zerit XR
Skin Effects: none noted

tenofovir disoproxil fumarate This medication is used for the treatment of HIV. It is commonly used with other medications.

Side Effects: upset stomach, changes in appetite, diarrhea, vomiting
Trade Name: Viread
Skin Effects: none noted

zalcitabine This medication is used to treat HIV and AIDS.

Side Effects: headache, fatigue, or fever, neuropathy in the arms and legs
Trade Name: HIVID
Skin Effects: ulcers in the mouth

zidovudine This medication is used in combination with other medications to treat HIV/AIDS.

Side Effects: headache, stomach pain, diarrhea, nausea, anemia, granulocytopenia
Trade Names: AZT, Retrovir
Skin Effects: nail pigmentation

Protease Inhibitors

These medications actually interfere with the reproduction of the virus.

amprenavir This drug is used to treat HIV. It is a protease inhibitor that slows the spread of the virus.

Side Effects: depression and mood changes, diarrhea, nausea, changes in taste, vomiting, **hyperglycemia**, **hyperlipidemia**
Trade Name: Agenerase
Skin Effects: rash

hyperglycemia
increased blood sugar levels often leading to diabetic coma if unresolved

hyperlipidemia
abnormally high levels of fat in the blood

atazanavir This medication is used for the treatment of HIV.

Side Effects: nausea, headache, depression, changes in sleep, redistribution of fat
Trade Name: Reyataz
Skin Effects: rash

fosamprenavir calcium This medication is used for the treatment of HIV and is used with other antivirals.

Side Effects: headache, diarrhea, nausea, vomiting
Trade Name: Lexiva
Skin Effects: rash

indinavir This medication is used to treat HIV.

Side Effects: dizziness, fatigue, diarrhea, nausea, vomiting, nephrolithiasis, redistribution of body fat

Trade Name: Crixivan
Skin Effects: none noted

lopinavir/ritonavir This medication is used for the treatment of HIV.

Side Effects: diarrhea, changes in taste
Trade Name: Kaletra
Skin Effects: rashes

nelfinavir mesylate This is an antiviral agent used for the treatment of HIV.

Side Effects: diarrhea
Trade Name: Viracept
Skin Effects: itching, rash, sweating, hives

ritonavir This medication is used for the treatment of HIV.

Side Effects: anxiety, depression, rhinitis, diarrhea, anorexia, dehydration
Trade Name: Norvir
Skin Effects: itching, rash, sweating, hives

saquinavir This medication is used in combination with other agents for the treatment of HIV.

Side Effects: abdominal pain, diarrhea, increased liver enzymes
Trade Name: Invirase
Skin Effects: yellow color to the skin, photosensitivity, severe cutaneous reactions such as Stevens-Johnson syndrome

tipranavir This medication is used for the treatment of advanced HIV.

Side Effects: increased lipids
Trade Name: Aptivus
Skin Effects: rashes, especially in women

Fusion Inhibitors

This medication is given subcutaneously and works by disallowing the cellular membrane to fuse.

enfuvirtide

Side Effects: fatigue, diarrhea, nausea
Trade Name: Fuzeon
Skin Effects: irritation at injection sites

Conclusion

Antiviral drugs are an important line of defense against many serious or recurrent viruses. As an aesthetician, you need to know which conditions your client has and what medications your client is taking for them. Because many of the treatments you will be performing cause injury to the skin, patients who have a latent virus may be subject to a recurrent infection. This is especially true of the herpes virus. Additionally, long term viral infections such as HIV or hepatitis B may have implications for the skin that should be researched separately under the specific disease.

REFERENCES

1. http://www.nlm.nih.gov
2. http://www.rxlist.com
3. http://www.drugs.com
4. Deglin, J. H., & Vallerand, A. H. (2007) *Davis's Drug Guide for Nurses.* Philadelphia, PA: F. A. Davis.
5. Michalun, N. (2001). *Milady's Skin Care and Cosmetic Ingredients Dictionary.* Clifton Park: Thomson Delmar Learning.
6. Spratto, G. R., & Woods, A. L. (2005). *2005 PDR Nurse's Drug Handbook.* Clifton Park: Thomson Delmar Learning.
7. http://www.fda.gov

Antifungals

CHAPTER 12

KEY TERMS

Athlete's Foot
Epidermal Necrolysis
Immunocompromised
Nephrotoxicity
Onychomycosis
Opportunistic Mycoses
Pathogenic Fungi
Subcutaneous Mycoses
Superficial Mycoses
Systemic Antifungals
Systemic Mycoses
Tinea Capitis
Tinea Corporis
Tinea Cruris
Topical Antifungals

LEARNING OBJECTIVES

After completing this chapter, you should be able to:

1. Explain the nature of fungal infections.
2. Identify some of the more common cutaneous fungal infections.
3. List some of the topical drugs that are used to treat fungal infections.
4. List some of the systemic drugs that are used to treat fungal infections.

INTRODUCTION

Fungal infections usually occur in darker, moister areas of the body, often where skin surfaces join together, for example, where the toes meet the trunk of the feet. Fungi are a species of parasite that feed from their hosts and reproduce both sexually and asexually.

pathogenic fungi
any fungus that results in disease

superficial mycoses
usually result from the introduction of vegetative matter to an open wound; infection is limited to the dermis

subcutaneous mycoses
a fungus that occurs under the skin

systemic mycoses
a fungus that affects the internal organs

opportunistic mycoses
any fungus that uses discontinuations in the skin or abnormal immunity to infect the body

immunocompromised
referring to limited or reduced functioning of the immune system

Pathogenic fungi, or fungi that cause or are a result of disease, are also known as mycoses and are classified according to the depth to which they invade the skin. **Superficial mycoses** are the most common and are localized to the exterior layers of the dermis in the skin and its appendages. The fungi live and produce in the area of infection. These include tineas and ringworm. **Subcutaneous mycoses** are rare, occurring mostly in tropical regions, and usually result from the introduction of vegetative matter to an open wound. Like superficial mycoses, the infection is limited to the dermis. They tend to have a slow onset and are chronic. **Systemic mycoses** are equally rare and affect the internal organs. **Opportunistic mycoses** usually occur in **immunocompromised** patients such as one who is undergoing chemotherapy or one who has just undergone surgery. These infections can be localized, or they can spread throughout the body. These infections can sometimes be fatal.

COMMON FUNGAL INFECTIONS

Our bodies contain natural flora that are harmless, and often vital, to overall bodily health. However, there are some fungi that can cause a fungal infection of the skin. These fungi can spread easily from one person to the next. The associated infections are generally not considered to be serious conditions and are typically easily remedied. However, rare

Table 12-1 Types of Fungal Mycoses

Type of Mycoses	Description
Superficial mycoses	Localized to the exterior layers of the dermis in the skin and its appendages
Subcutaneous mycoses	Usually result from the introduction of vegetative matter to an open wound; infection is limited to the dermis
Systemic mycoses	Affect the internal organs
Opportunistic mycoses	Occur in immunocompromised patients

Table 12-2 Causes for Fungal Infections
A course of antibiotics recently taken
Immune system weakened by cancer or HIV infection
Oral steroids taken
Diabetic
Moist skin or humid environs
Exposed cuts or wounds

systemic mycoses can be more problematic. The symptoms and appearances of a fungal skin infection depend on the type of fungus causing it and the part of the body affected. Usually, the fungal infections will present with a rash. Different types of fungal infections are usually named for the part of the body in which they present.

The rash may have a variety of appearances. Some rashes are red, scaly, and itchy, whereas others can produce a fine scale similar to dry skin. The site of infection may be just one area of the body, or there may be several infected areas.

Athlete's foot is a common infection and is often caused by a combination of fungi and bacteria. It causes scaling and sogginess of the skin, commonly of the web spaces between the toes. Sometimes the skin becomes pale and can be itchy. Infection is often picked up from contaminated skin fragments in public places, such as swimming pools and shower facilities.

Onychomycosis is the name for any fungal nail infection. Tinea unguium (ringworm of the nails) is a common one. The nails become malformed, thickened, and crumbly. Not all nails affected like this are caused by fungal infections, but it is a common cause. Toenail infections are commonly linked with athlete's foot. Fingernails can be affected, too.

Tinea cruris is called "jock itch" because it occurs in sportspeople. It causes an itchy, red rash in the groin and surrounding area and is commonly seen in men who have been sweating a lot. Often the man also has athlete's foot, and scratching the feet followed by touching or scratching the groin may spread the infection.

Tinea corporis or ringworm affects the body, often in exposed areas, by causing red patches, which are scaly at the edge with clear skin at the center. The patches spread out from the center. It can be caught from domestic animals.

Tinea capitis is ringworm of the scalp and tends to affect young children. It can cause hair loss with inflammation in the affected area.

athlete's foot
contagious fungal infection of the feet (aka tinea pedis)

onychomycosis
parasitic infection of the nails

tinea cruris
fungal infection of the area surrounding the genitalia (aka jock itch)

tinea corporis
fungal infection of the skin on the body (aka ringworm)

tinea capitis
fungal infection of the scalp

Systemic Antifungals

systemic antifungals
antifungal medications that are ingested and distributed via the bloodstream

nephrotoxicity
kidney toxicity

Systemic antifungals are medications that are used orally or intravenously to manage fungal infections.

amphotericin B deoxycholate This antifungal is used to treat serious, potentially fatal fungus infections.

Side Effects: headache, low blood pressure, diarrhea, nausea, vomiting, **nephrotoxicity**, hypokalemia, chills, fever
Trade Name: Fungizone
Skin Effects: none noted

amphotericin B cholesteryl sulfate

Side Effects: headache, low blood pressure, diarrhea, nausea, vomiting, nephrotoxicity, hypokalemia, chills, fever
Trade Name: Amphotec
Skin Effects: none noted

amphotericin B lipid complex

Side Effects: headache, low blood pressure, diarrhea, nausea, vomiting, nephrotoxicity, hypokalemia, chills, fever
Trade Name: Abelcet
Skin Effects: none noted

amphotericin B liposome

Side Effects: headache, low blood pressure, diarrhea, nausea, vomiting, nephrotoxicity, hypokalemia, chills, fever
Trade Name: AmBisome
Skin Effects: none noted

caspofungin This product is used intravenously for the treatment of fungal infections.

Side Effects: side effects are rare with this medication
Trade Name: Cancidas
Skin Effects: flushing

fluconazole This drug is used to treat fungal infections any place in the body, including mouth, vagina, esophagus, lungs, blood, or other organs.

Side Effects: Side effects are rare with this medication
Trade Name: Diflucan
Skin Effects: exfoliative skin disorders, Stevens-Johnson syndrome

itraconazole This medication is used for the treatment of fungal infections in the fingernails, toenails, and esophagus.

Side Effects: nausea
Trade Name: Sporanox
Skin Effects: rash, itching, toxic **epidermal necrolysis,** and photosensitivity

epidermal necrolysis tissue death on the epidermis

topical antifungals any antifungal medication that is applied on top of the skin

ketoconazole This drug is used to treat fungal infections that can spread through the body. This drug can also be used to treat fungal infections in the nails and skin.

Side Effects: nausea
Trade Name: Nizoral
Skin Effects: rash

terbinafine This drug is used to manage fungal infections of the nails.

Side Effects: diarrhea, nausea, vomiting, stomach pain, anorexia
Trade Name: Lamisil
Skin Effects: rash or itching, toxic epidermal necrolysis

voriconazole This medication is used to manage more serious fungal infections, including those of the esophagus, skin, abdomen, kidney, and bladder, as well as those fungal infections found in wounds accompanied by bacterial infections.

Side Effects: changes in vision
Trade Name: VFEND
Skin Effects: rash, photosensitivity

Topical Antifungals

Topical antifungals are those medications that are applied to the skin for the management of a fungal infection.

butenafine This medication is used to manage fungal infections. It is applied topically to the affected area. It is useful for athlete's foot, tinea cruris, tinea corporis, and tinea versicolor.

Side Effects: no noted systemic side effects
Trade Name: Lotrimin Ultra, Mentax
Skin Effects: burning, itching, hypersensitivity at the site of application, redness, stinging

butoconazole This drug is used to manage vaginal yeast infections.

Side Effects: headache, stomachache, fever, or odorous discharge from the vagina
Trade Name: Gynazole-1
Skin Effects: burning, irritation

ciclopirox This medication is used to manage fungal infections. It is applied topically to the affected area. It is useful for athlete's foot, tinea cruris, tinea corporis, and tinea versicolor.

Side Effects: no noted systemic side effects
Trade Names: Loprox, Penlac
Skin Effects: burning, itching, hypersensitivity at the site of application, redness, stinging

clotrimazole This drug is used to treat yeast infections. These infections are commonly found in the vagina, in the mouth, and on the skin.

Side Effects: stomachache, nausea, vomiting, fever
Trade Names: Lotrimin, Mycelex, Mycelex OTC
Skin Effects: burning, itching, hypersensitivity at the site of application, redness, stinging

econazole This product is used to treat ringworm, jock itch, and athlete's foot.

Side Effects: no systemic effects were noted
Trade Name: Spectazole
Skin Effects: burning, itching, hypersensitivity at the site of application, redness, stinging

haloprogin This medication is used to manage fungal infections. It is applied topically to the affected area. It is useful for athlete's foot, tinea cruris, tinea corporis, and tinea versicolor.

Side Effects: no systemic effects were noted
Trade Name: Halotex
Skin Effects: burning, itching, hypersensitivity at the site of application, redness, stinging

ketoconazole This medication is used to manage fungal infections. It is applied topically to the affected area. It is useful for athlete's foot, tinea cruris, tinea corporis, and tinea versicolor.

Side Effects: no systemic effects were noted
Trade Name: Nizoral
Skin Effects: burning, itching, hypersensitivity at the site of application, redness, stinging

miconazole This medication is used to manage fungal infections. It is applied topically to the affected area. It is useful for athlete's foot, tinea cruris, tinea corporis, and tinea versicolor.

Side Effects: stomach pain, fever, pungent vaginal discharge
Trade Names: Breezee Mist Antifungal, Fungoid, Micatin, Monistat-Derm, Ony-Clear, Tetterine
Skin Effects: burning, itching, hypersensitivity at the site of application, redness, stinging

naftifine This product is used for fungal infections such as athlete's foot, jock itch, and ringworm.

Side Effects: no systemic symptoms are noted
Trade Name: Naftin
Skin Effects: rash, dryness, burning, itching, stinging, redness.

nystatin This product is used for fungal infections such as athlete's foot, jock itch, and ringworm.

Side Effects: no systemic symptoms are noted
Trade Names: Mycostatin, Nystex, Pedi-Dri
Skin Effects: rash, dryness, burning, itching, stinging, redness.

oxiconazole An antifungal product used for athlete's foot, jock itch, and ringworm.

Side Effects: no systemic symptoms are noted
Trade Name: Oxistat
Skin Effects: rash, dryness, burning, itching, stinging, redness.

sertaconazole This medication is used for the treatment in pediatric tinea pedis.

Side Effects: none noted
Trade Name: Ertaczo
Skin Effects: none noted

sulconazole This medication is used for the treatment of fungal infections.

Side Effects: no systemic side effects were noted
Trade Name: Exelderm
Skin Effects: redness or burning can occur where the medication is placed. Also, rashes, itching, stinging, and irritation are possible.

terconazole This product is used to manage yeast and fungal infections of the vagina.

Side Effects: headache, changes in menstrual cycles, stomach pain or fever, a pungent discharge from the vagina.
Trade Name: Terazol
Skin Effects: burning, irritation.

terbinafine This drug is used to manage fungal infections of the nails.

Side Effects: anorexia, diarrhea, nausea, stomach pain, vomiting
Trade Name: Lamisil
Skin Effects: rash or itching, hives, toxic epidermal necrolysis

tioconazole This medication is used for the treatment of vaginal fungal infections.

Side Effects: headache
Trade Name: Vagistat
Skin Effects: local irritation, sensitization, vulvovaginal burning

tolnaftate An antifungal product used for athlete's foot, jock itch, and ringworm.

Side Effects: none noted
Trade Names: Aftate, Dr. Scholl's Athlete's Foot Cream, Dr. Scholl's Maximum Strength Tritan, Quinsana Plus, Tinactin, Ting
Skin Effects: burning, itching, local sensitivity, redness, stinging

Conclusion

Fungus infections typically find a place to grow on the human skin or in the human lung. Because of an increased use of broad-spectrum antibiotics, immunosuppressive agents, AIDS, organ transplants, and medications used in the hospital setting, systemic fungal infections are more common than they used to be. The structure and chemical makeup of a fungus can make it difficult to treat. Consequently, there are many antifungal drugs available, some of which are topical and the others systemic.

REFERENCES

1. Deglin, J. H., & Vallerand, A. H. (2007). *Davis's Drug Guide for Nurses.* Philadelphia, PA: F. A. Davis.
2. Lesher, J., & Woody, C. M. (2003). Antimicrobial Drugs. In J. Bolognia, J. Jorizzo, & R. Rapini (Eds.), *Dermatology* (pp. 2007–2031). Philadelphia, PA: Mosby.

CHAPTER 13

Antineoplastics

KEY TERMS

Bronchogenic Cancers
Desquamation
Electrolytes
Endometrium
Erythema Nodosum
Hand and Foot Syndrome
Hepatic Transaminases
Hodgkin's Disease
Hyperuricemia
Kaposi's Sarcoma
Leukemias
Leukopenia
Lymphocytic Leukemia
Maculopapular
Metastatic
Mucocutaneous Toxicity
Mucositis
Multiple Myeloma
Mycosis Fungoides
Myelogenous
Nephropathy
Neuroblastoma
Non-Hodgkin's Lymphoma
Oliguria
Palmar-Plantar Erythrodysesthesia
Pleural Effusion
Pneumonitis
Rigors
Thrombocytopekopenia
Thrombocytopenia

LEARNING OBJECTIVES

After completing this chapter, you should be able to:

1. Understand the different means of treating cancer.
2. Define chemotherapy.
3. Define the drugs used to treat cancer.

INTRODUCTION TO DRUGS USED TO TREAT CANCER

Cancer is one of the leading causes of death for Americans. Researchers have sought for the elusive cure for cancer, but have been unsuccessful thus far. This is because there exist many types of cancer, and it is thought that there may be hundred of thousands of carcinogens in our environment. With so many carcinogens causing so many types of cancer, the task of finding a cure is daunting. While a cure is pursued, a variety of drugs are available to treat cancer. These drugs are called antineoplastics.

There are currently three ways to attack cancer: chemotherapy, radiation, and surgery. Any drug that is used to treat cancer is referred to as a chemotherapy agent. Because the subject manner of this text is drugs, emphasis will be placed on chemotherapy.

Antineoplastics are very powerful medications that operate in a variety of ways, and there are several drawbacks to these drugs. There are several reasons that the development of antineoplastic drugs has proven to be challenging for the scientist. Cancer cells are biochemically similar to normal cells; therefore, it is difficult to create an antineoplastic drug that will not harm normal cells. The second problem is that even the drugs that effectively target the correct chemical markers in cancer cells seem to be highly toxic to other normal cell producing mechanisms of the body, for instance, bone marrow. Finally, anticancer drugs that inhibit cancerous cell production have only a limited efficacy. Toxicity is common. For this reason cancer chemotherapy may consist of using several drugs in combination for varying lengths of time.

Further complicating matters, other drugs are used to treat cancer but are not usually considered to be "chemotherapy." While chemotherapy drugs take advantage of the fact that cancer cells divide rapidly, these other drugs target rare properties that set certain cancer cells apart from normal cells. They often have less serious side effects than those commonly caused by chemotherapy drugs.

Chemotherapy

As mentioned above, anticancer drugs are collectively called chemotherapy drugs or antineoplastics. Antineoplastics are divided into several categories, which are determined by how they affect specific chemical substances within cancer cells. Chemotherapy drugs work to accomplish several tasks, all aimed at slowing or, ideally, halting cancer cell growth by hindering the replication of their DNA. To this effect, antineoplastics take advantage of the rapid replication of cancer cells. Consequently, they also have side effects for other bodily systems that utilize rapid cell replication, such as hair growth, white cell production, and skin building. Types of chemotherapy subgroups include alkylating agents, anthracyclines, antiandrogens, antiestrogens, antimetabolites, antitumor antibiotics, aromatase inhibitors, enzymes, hormones, monoclonal antibodies, podophyllotoxin derivatives, progestins, taxoids, vinca alkaloids, and other miscellaneous drugs.

Alkylating Agents

Alkylating agents are a class of drugs that operate by preventing DNA replication within cancer cells. Alkylating agents attach methyl or other alkyl groups onto molecules where they do not belong, resulting in damage to the DNA of the individual cancer cells. These drugs are used to treat several types of cancer, including chronic **leukemias**, **non-Hodgkin's lymphoma**, **Hodgkin's disease**, and **multiple myeloma**, as well as lung, breast, and ovarian cancers.

leukemia
a malignant cancer of the blood producing tissues

non-Hodgkin's lymphoma
a certain type of malignant cancer originating in the lymphatic system

Hodgkin's disease
malignant tumor of the lymph system

multiple myeloma
malignant neoplastic condition characterized by tumor cells infiltrating the bone and bone marrow

myelogenous
originating in the bone marrow

oliguria
lessening in the amount of urine

erythema nodosum
characterized by tender, red bumps, usually found on the shins. Quite often, erythema nodosum is not a separate disease, but, rather, a sign of some other disease, or of a sensitivity to a drug

electrolytes
any solution that conducts electricity in the body, most commonly salts, potassium, and chlorine

Antineoplastics

busulfan This drug is used for the treatment of chronic **myelogenous** (myeloid, myelocytic, granulocytic) leukemia.

Side Effects: anxiety, confusion, depression, dizziness, headache, weakness, nosebleeds, pharyngitis, chest pain, low blood pressure, fast heartbeat, blood clots, abdominal enlargement, anorexia, constipation, diarrhea, dry mouth, vomiting blood, nausea, vomiting, rectal pain, **oliguria,** hyperglycemia, arthralgia, myalgia, allergic reactions, fever, chills, infections
Trade Names: Busulfex, Myleran
Skin Effects: itching, rashes, acne, alopecia, **erythema nodosum**, exfoliative dermatitis, hyperpigmentation

carboplatin This drug is used to treat cancer of the ovaries; it is given only intravenously.

Side Effects: nausea, vomiting, abdominal pain, tiredness and weakness, changes in bowel habits, loss of appetite, changes in **electrolytes**
Trade Name: Paraplatin
Skin Effects: alopecia, rashes

carmustine This drug is used to treat the following types of cancer: brain tumors, multiple myeloma, Hodgkin's disease, non-Hodgkin's lymphoma.

Side Effects: liver toxicity, nausea, vomiting

Trade Names: BiCNU, BCNU, Gliadel
Skin Effects: alopecia

chlorambucil This drug is used in the treatment of chronic **lymphocytic leukemia**, some types of non-Hodgkin's lymphomas, and advanced Hodgkin's disease.

Side Effects: **hyperuricemia**
Trade Name: Leukeran
Skin Effects: alopecia, dermatitis, rashes

cisplatin This drug is used for advanced bladder cancer, spreading testicular cancers, spreading ovarian cancers, head and neck cancers, cervical cancers, and lung cancers and is given only intravenously.

Side Effects: toxic effect on hearing, ringing in the ears, nausea, vomiting, changes in electrolytes, anemia
Trade Name: Platinol-AQ
Skin Effects: alopecia

cyclophosphamide This drug is used to treat Hodgkin's disease, lymphomas, multiple myeloma, leukemias, **mycosis fungoides, neuroblastoma,** ovarian carcinoma, retinoblastoma, and breast cancer.

Side Effects: anorexia, nausea, vomiting, blood in the urine, changes in the blood count
Trade Names: Cytoxan, Neosar
Skin Effects: alopecia

ifosfamide This drug treats cancer of the testis.

Side Effects: central nervous system toxicity, nausea, vomiting, bleeding from the bladder
Trade Name: IFEX
Skin Effects: alopecia

melphalan This drug is used to treat multiple myeloma and ovarian cancer.

Side Effects: **leukopenia, thrombocytopenia**
Trade Names: Alkeran, L-PAM, phenylalanine mustard
Skin Effects: skin hypersensitivities, alopecia, rashes, itching

mechlorethamine This drug is used for Hodgkin's disease and malignant lymphomas and is given intravenously.

Side Effects: nausea, vomiting, anemia

lymphocytic leukemia
a form of childhood cancer

hyperuricemia
abnormally high levels of uric acid in the blood

mycosis fungoides
a rare T-cell skin cancer

neuroblastoma
a certain type of malignant tumor originating in neuroblast cells of the brain

leukopenia
unusual decrease in white blood cells

thrombocytopenia
abnormal decrease in blood platelet levels

Trade Names: Mustargen, nitrogen mustard
Skin Effects: alopecia, rashes

procarbazine This drug is used in combination with other anticancer drugs in the treatment of Stage III and Stage IV Hodgkin's disease.

Side Effects: nausea, vomiting, **pleural effusion**, cough, edema, confusion
Trade Name: Matulane
Skin Effects: pruritus, alopecia, rashes, photosensitivity

pleural effusion
fluid leakage in the thoracic cavity

Kaposi's sarcoma
condition characterized by multiple areas of cell proliferation that eventually become cancerous

bronchogenic cancers
lung cancer that originates in the bronchus

temozolomide This medicine is used to treat brain cancer.

Side Effects: nausea, vomiting, headache, leukopenia, thrombocytopenia
Trade Name: Temodar
Skin Effects: itching, rashes

Anthracyclines

Like other anticancer drugs, anthracyclines disrupt DNA replication. They are technically considered antibiotics; however, they are rarely used as such. Their anticancerous qualities render them useful to chemotherapy though. They are used to treat a wide variety of cancers, particularly leukemia. However, they can have a negative effect on heart muscle.

daunorubicin citrate liposome This drug is used to treat **Kaposi's sarcoma** and is given intravenously.

Side Effects: fatigue, headache, rhinitis, changes in the color of urine, anemia, leukopenia, thrombocytopenia, pain, neuropathy, allergic responses, chills, fever, flushing, tight chest
Trade Name: DaunoXome
Skin Effects: alopecia, sweating, itching

daunorubicin hydrochloride This drug is used in the treatment of leukemia and is given intravenously.

Side Effects: rhinitis, nausea, vomiting, changes in the color of urine, anemia, leukopenia, thrombocytopenia, phlebitis at the IV site
Trade Name: Cerubidine
Skin Effects: alopecia

doxorubicin hydrochloride This drug is used to treat cancers of the breast, ovaries, and bladder, as well as **bronchogenic cancers**, lymphomas, and leukemia. It is given intravenously.

Side Effects: diarrhea, esophagitis, nausea, stomatitis, vomiting, red urine, anemia, leukopenia, thrombocytopenia, phlebitis at IV site
Trade Names: Adriamycin PFS, Adriamycin RDF, Rubex
Skin Effects: alopecia, photosensitivity

doxorubicin hydrochloride liposome This drug is used for **metastatic** ovarian cancer and AIDS related Kaposi's sarcoma.

Side Effects: nausea, anemia, leukopenia, thrombocytopenia
Trade Name: Doxil
Skin Effects: alopecia, **palmar-plantar erythrodysesthesia**

epirubicin This drug is used for the treatment of breast cancer and is given intravenously.

Side Effects: nausea, vomiting
Trade Name: Ellence
Skin Effects: alopecia

idarubicin This drug is used for treating leukemia and is given intravenously.

Side Effects: headache, changes in mental status, pulmonary toxicity, abdominal cramps, diarrhea, **mucositis**, nausea, vomiting, anemia, leukopenia, thrombocytopenia, fever, phlebitis at IV site
Trade Name: Idamycin
Skin Effects: alopecia, rashes, photosensitivity

metastatic
movement of bacterial or cancer cells from one part of the body to another

palmar-plantar erythrodysesthesia
condition characterized by redness and pain on the palm and soles of the feet

mucositis
inflammation of the mucous membranes

Antiandrogens

Androgens are the male sex hormone testosterone. Antiandrogens work to block the receptors on the cell's surface, preventing the androgens' pathway. These medications are given to treat prostate cancer.

bicalutamide This drug treats prostate cancer.

Side Effects: weakness, diarrhea, constipation, nausea
Trade Name: Casodex
Skin Effects: alopecia, rashes, sweating

flutamide This drug is used for the treatment of prostate cancer.

Side Effects: hot flashes, diarrhea, nausea, vomiting, impotence, loss of sexual drive, enlargement of the breasts

Trade Name: Eulexin
Skin Effects: skin rashes, photosensitivity

nilutamide This drug is used to treat prostate cancer.

Side Effects: inability to adapt to darkness
Trade Name: Nilandron
Skin Effects: hot flashes, alopecia, sweating

Antiestrogens

This group of medications is used to treat tumors that are estrogen dependent. They are typically used to treat breast cancer, an estrogen dependent tumor. Antiestrogens work by blocking the protein to the cancer cell.

tamoxifen This drug is used to treat breast cancer in both women and men. Other uses may include treatment of malignant melanoma and cancer of the **endometrium.**

endometrium
the mucous membrane lining the interior walls of the uterus

Side Effects: nausea, vomiting
Trade Name: Nolvadex
Skin Effects: none noted

toremifene This drug is used in the treatment of breast cancer that is spreading.

Side Effects: nausea, vaginal discharge
Trade Name: Fareston
Skin Effects: hot flashes, sweating

Antimetabolites

Antimetabolites are a category of anticancer drugs that inhibit DNA growth. They accomplish this in a "Trojan horse" manner. Metabolites, the general name for organic compounds that are broken down and used by the body, are structurally similar to antimetabolites (so much so that the cancer cells cannot tell any difference). The difference is that they cannot be used in any way. By inserting the Trojan horse antimetabolites, the cancer cells cannot replicate. Antimetabolites are used to treat a variety of cancers, including leukemias, breast cancer, ovarian cancer, cancers of the gastrointestinal tract, as well as other cancers.

capecitabine This drug is used to treat colorectal cancer and breast cancer.

Side Effects: diarrhea, nausea, vomiting, fatigue, headache, eye irritation, swelling, abdominal pain, anorexia, constipation, increased

bilirubin, changes in taste, stomatitis, muscle pain, joint pain, cough, shortness of breath
Trade Name: Xeloda
Skin Effects: **hand and foot syndrome**, dermatitis, nail disorders, alopecia, erythema, rashes

hand and foot syndrome
condition characterized by painful lesions on the hands and feet

maculopapular
eruptions of both macules and papules

hepatic transaminases
a type of liver enzyme

cytarabine This drug is used in the treatment of leukemia and non-Hodgkin's lymphomas and is given intravenously.

Side Effects: nausea, vomiting, anemia, leukopenia, thrombocytopenia
Trade Names: Ara-C, cytosine arabinoside, Cytosar-U, DepoCyt
Skin Effects: alopecia, rashes

fluorouracil This drug treats cancer of the breast, rectum, colon, stomach, and pancreas. It is also used topically to treat actinic (solar) keratoses and basal cell carcinoma.

Side Effects: loss of appetite, nausea, vomiting, weakness, diarrhea, stomatitis, anemia, leukopenia, thrombocytopenia
Trade Names: Adrucil, Efudex, Fluoroplex, 5-FU
Skin Effects: alopecia, **maculopapular** rash, local inflammatory reactions, pigment in the nails, nail loss, palmar-plantar erythrodysesthesia, phototoxicity

gemcitabine hydrochloride This drug is used for the treatment of adenocarcinoma of the pancreas, breast cancer, and certain types of lung cancer. It is given intravenously.

Side Effects: dyspnea, diarrhea, edema, nausea, stomatitis, transient elevation of **hepatic transaminases,** vomiting, hematuria, proteinuria, anemia, leukopenia, thrombocytopenia, flu-like symptoms
Trade Name: Gemzar
Skin Effects: alopecia, rashes

hydroxyurea This drug is used for head and neck cancer, ovarian cancers, and sickle cell anemia.

Side Effects: anorexia, diarrhea, nausea, vomiting, leukopenia
Trade Name: Hydrea
Skin Effects: alopecia, erythema, pruritus, rashes

methotrexate This drug is used to treat cancer of the breast, head and neck, lung, blood, bone, and lymph, as well as tumors in the uterus.

nephropathy
kidney disease

desquamation
normal sloughing of the epidermis

pneumonitis
inflammation of the lungs

mucocutaneous toxicity
poisoning of the skin and mucous membranes

Side Effects: loss of appetite, nausea, vomiting, liver toxicity, stomatitis, anemia, leukopenia, thrombocytopenia, **nephropathy**
Trade Names: amethopterin, Folex, Folex PFS, Rheumatrex, Trexall
Skin Effects: alopecia, photosensitivity, rashes, pruritus, skin ulcers, hives

pemetrexed This drug is used to treat specific types of lung cancers, and it is given intravenously.

Side Effects: inflammation of the pharynx, constipation, nausea, vomiting, stomatitis, fever, infection
Trade Name: Alimta
Skin Effects: **desquamation,** rashes

Antitumor antibiotics

A key step in the survival of the cell is the production of RNA, which produces protein in the cell. All cells need protein to live. Antitumor antibiotics interfere with the synthesis of RNA and as such cell reproduction. These antitumor antibiotics are not the same type of antibiotic used to treat infections. Rather than fight infection, these antibiotics cause the DNA to malfunction and prevent the RNA production of protein.

bleomycin sulfate This drug is used to treat lymphoma, squamous cell carcinoma, and testicular cancers.

Side Effects: chills, fever, **pneumonitis**
Trade Name: Blenoxane
Skin Effects: hyperpigmentation, **mucocutaneous toxicity**, alopecia, erythema, rashes, hives, vesiculation

mitomycin This drug is used to treat cancers of the stomach and pancreas, and it is given intravenously.

Side Effects: nausea, vomiting, leukopenia, thrombocytopenia, phlebitis
Trade Names: MitoExtra, Mutamycin
Skin Effects: alopecia, desquamation

mitoxantrone This drug is used to treat prostate cancer, leukemia, and multiple sclerosis.

Side Effects: headache, cough, shortness of breath, abdominal pain, diarrhea, liver toxicity, nausea, stomatitis, vomiting, anemia, leukopenia, thrombocytopekopenia, fever
Trade Name: Novantrone
Skin Effects: alopecia, rashes

Aromatase inhibitors

Tumors that are estrogen sensitive require estrogen to grow. Typically these tumors are in the breast or ovaries. Aromatase inhibitors help to block the production of estrogen in the body.

anastrazole This medication is used in the treatment of breast cancer, typically breast cancer that is spreading throughout the body.

Side Effects: headache, weakness, nausea, back pain, hot flashes, pain
Trade Name: Arimidex
Skin Effects: rashes, mucocutaneous disorders, sweating

letrozole This medication is used to treat advanced breast cancer.

Side Effects: pain in the muscles and bones
Trade Name: Femara
Skin Effects: alopecia, hot flashes, sweating, itching, rashes

Enzyme Inhibitors

Enzymes are important in the daily functioning of the body. Drugs that inhibit the functioning of an enzyme and prevent it from functioning are called enzyme inhibitors. For example, poisons are also enzyme inhibitors.

erlotinib This drug is used in the treatment of advanced or spreading lung cancers.

Side Effects: diarrhea, shortness of breath
Trade Name: Tarceva
Skin Effects: rashes, dry skin, itching

gefitinib This drug is used to treat certain types of lung cancer.

Side Effects: diarrhea, nausea, vomiting
Trade Name: Iressa
Skin Effects: acne, dry skin, rashes, itching

imatinib This drug is used in the treatment of leukemia gastrointestinal stomach tumors.

Side Effects: fatigue, headache, weakness, cough, shortness of breath, nosebleeds, nasopharyngitis, pneumonia, stomach pain, anorexia, constipation, diarrhea, upset stomach, nausea, vomiting, swelling, weight gain, joint pain, muscle pain and cramps, bone pain, fever, night sweats

Trade Name: Gleevec
Skin Effects: rashes, red dots on the skin, itching

irinotecan This drug is used for cancer that is spreading from the colon and rectum. This drug is given intravenously.

Side Effects: dizziness, headache, coughing, difficulty breathing, inflammation of the nose, nausea, vomiting, diarrhea, pain, fever, swelling, vasodilation, constipation, anorexia, abdominal pain, upset stomach, gas, stomatitis, anemia, dehydration, weight loss, back pain, chills
Trade Name: Camptosar
Skin Effects: rashes, alopecia, sweating

topotecan This drug is used to treat ovarian cancer and lung cancers. This drug is given intravenously.

Side Effects: headache, nausea, vomiting, diarrhea, abdominal pain, loss of appetite, constipation, shortness of breath
Trade Name: Hycamtin
Skin Effects: alopecia

Enzymes

Enzymes are proteins that speed up chemical reactions. Enzyme activity can be influenced by specific factors. The specific activity of an enzyme is determined by its structure. In the case of cancer treatment, enzymes are used to inhibit the growth of the tumor.

asparaginase This drug is used to treat leukemia, and this medication is given intravenously.

Side Effects: nausea, vomiting
Trade Name: Elspar
Skin Effects: skin rashes, hives

pegaspargase This medication is used to treat leukemia and is given intravenously.

Side Effects: side effects are not common
Trade Names: Oncaspar, PEG-L-asparaginase
Skin Effects: jaundice

Hormones

Hormones are naturally occurring or synthetic hormones that are structurally similar to steroids. They are used therapeutically to mimic or augment the effects of the naturally occurring hormones, which are produced in the cortex of the adrenal gland. Hormones are very powerful drugs that affect the entire body; even corticosteroids used on large areas of skin for long periods are absorbed in sufficient quantity to cause systemic effects. They are themselves a specific drug category; however, when used to treat cancer they are considered a chemotherapy agent. They are useful in treating some types of cancer, including lymphoma, leukemia, and multiple myeloma.

goserelin acetate This drug is used to treat breast cancer and prostate cancer, and this medication is given subcutaneously.

Side Effects: headache, vasodilation, impotence, bone pain, hot flashes
Trade Name: Zoladex
Skin Effects: sweating, rashes

leuprolide This medication is used to treat advanced prostate cancer, and it is given intramuscularly or subcutaneously or is implanted.

Side Effects: hot flashes
Trade Names: Eligard, Lupron, Lupron Depot, Lupron Depot–PED, Lupron Depot-3 Month, Viadur
Skin Effects: hair growth, rashes, dry skin, alopecia, pigmentation, skin cancer, skin lesions

medroxyprogesterone This drug is used to treat endometrial cancer and renal cancers.

Side Effects: side effects are not common
Trade Names: Amen, Curretab, Cycrin, Depo-Provera SubQ Provera 104, Provera
Skin Effects: chloasma, melasma, rashes

triptorelin This drug is used for treating prostate cancer.

Side Effects: changes in sexual function and desires, pain in the bones and muscles
Trade Names: Trelstar, Depot
Skin Effects: itching

Monoclonal Antibodies

This very high-tech drug category uses artificially produced proteins that bind to tissue antigens. These antibodies are derived from one cell, which makes them very specific. In fact, they are clones of the cell they are looking to obliterate. Drugs can be created to seek and destroy specific cancer cells.

alemtuzumab This drug treats leukemia, and it is given intravenously.

Side Effects: anemia, lymphopenia, thrombocytopenia
Trade Name: Campath
Skin Effects: rashes, sweating

bevacizumab This medication is used for colon and rectal cancers.

Side Effects: side effects are not common
Trade Name: Avastin
Skin Effects: none noted

cetuximab This drug is used for the treatment of colon and rectal cancers. This medication is given intravenously.

Side Effects: abdominal pain, constipation, diarrhea, nausea, vomiting, fever
Trade Name: Erbitux
Skin Effects: acne form of dermatitis, alopecia, nail disorders, itching, desquamation

gemtuzumab ozogamicin This drug is used to treat leukemia in patients 60 years of age and older, and it is given subcutaneously.

Side Effects: headache, vasodilation, changes in sexual desires, changes in sexual performance, bone pain, hot flashes
Trade Name: Mylotarg
Skin Effects: rashes, sweating

rituximab This drug is used to treat non-Hodgkin's lymphoma. This medication is administered intravenously.

rigors
hardness or stiffness of the muscles

Side Effects: low blood pressure, fever, chills, **rigors**
Trade Name: Rituxan
Skin Effects: flushing, hives, mucocutaneous skin reactions

trastuzumab This medication is used to treat breast cancers, and it is given intravenously.

Side Effects: abdominal pain, nausea, vomiting, diarrhea, anorexia, back pain, chills, fever, infection, generalized pain
Trade Name: Herceptin
Skin Effects: rashes, acne, herpes

Podophyllotoxin Derivatives

These synthetic drugs block the cell division of rapidly dividing cells, such as cancer cells.

etoposide This drug is used to treat lung cancer and testicular cancer, and it can be administered intravenously.

Side Effects: low blood pressure, nausea, vomiting, leukopenia, thrombocytopenia
Trade Names: VePesid, VP-16
Skin Effects: loss of hair

etoposide phosphate This drug is used to treat lung cancer and testicular cancer, and it can be administered intravenously.

Side Effects: low blood pressure, nausea, vomiting, leukopenia, thrombocytopenia
Trade Name: Etopophos
Skin Effects: loss of hair

Progestins

This drug has a progesterone effect and is used to treat endometrial cancers and breast cancers.

megestrol This drug is used to treat endometrial and breast cancers. It is also used in the treatment of anorexia in AIDS patients.

Side Effects: asymptomatic adrenal suppression
Trade Name: Megace
Skin Effects: alopecia

Taxoids

These semisynthetic medications are modeled on the natural substance taxol, which comes from yew trees found in the Pacific Northwest. The drug attaches to specific areas of the cell, preventing cell division. Because cancer cells divide more frequently than normal cells, these drugs attack the cell division, reducing the size of the tumor and slowing the progression of the disease.

docetaxel This medication is used to treat breast cancer that has spread, certain lung cancers, and prostate cancers, and it is given intravenously.

Side Effects: fatigue, weakness, swelling of the arms and legs, diarrhea, nausea, vomiting, stomatitis, anemia, thrombocytopenia, muscle pain
Trade Name: Taxotere
Skin Effects: alopecia, rashes, dermatitis, desquamation, skin swelling, erythema, nail disorders

paclitaxel This drug is used in the treatment of advanced ovarian cancer, breast cancer, and Kaposi's sarcoma, and it is given intravenously.

Side Effects: nausea, vomiting, diarrhea, anemia, leukopenia, thrombocytopenia, muscle pain, pain in the arms and legs
Trade Names: Onxol, Taxol
Possible Skin Effects: alopecia, maculopapular rashes, itching

Vinca Alkaloids

The category of vinca alkaloids works to treat cancer by preventing the cell division of the cancerous cell. In a complex process, the vinca alkaloids prevent the formation of mitotic spindles, which are necessary for DNA cells to divide. These drugs are derived from plants and administered intravenously.

vinblastine This medication is used to treat lymphomas, testicular cancers, and advanced breast cancer, and it is given intravenously.

Side Effects: nausea, vomiting, anemia, leukopenia, thrombocytopenia, phlebitis at the IV site
Trade Name: Velban
Skin Effects: alopecia, dermatitis, vesiculation

vincristine This drug is used for the treatment of acute leukemia, Hodgkin's disease, and non-Hodgkin's lymphoma, and it is given intravenously.

Side Effects: nausea, vomiting, numbness and tingling of the extremities, phlebitis at the site of injection
Trade Name: Oncovin
Skin Effects: alopecia

vinorelbine For the treatment of lung cancer, this drug is given intravenously.

Side Effects: nausea, constipation, fatigue, anemia, neutropenia, irritation at the IV site, neurotoxicity
Trade Name: Navelbine
Skin Effects: alopecia, rashes

Miscellaneous Anticancer Drugs

The following drugs have a variety of uses, from the treatment of prostate cancer to the treatment of colon and rectal cancer. Each one is specific to the disease process mentioned.

abarelix This drug is used for the treatment of prostate cancer and is given intramuscularly.

Side Effects: dizziness, fatigue, headache, sleep changes, swelling in the arms and legs, constipation, diarrhea, nausea, changes in urination, changes in the breast, possible swelling, back pain
Trade Name: Plenaxis
Skin Effects: hot flashes

aldesleukin This medication treats renal cancer that is spreading.

Side Effects: shortness of breath, pulmonary congestion, pulmonary edema, heartbeat irregularity, low blood pressure, fast heartbeat, diarrhea, nausea, vomiting, stomatitis, changes in the urine, changes in the electrolytes,
Trade Names: Proleukin, interleukin-2 IL-2
Skin Effects: exfolitative dermatitis, itching, yellow skin

alitretinoin This drug treats cutaneous lesions and Kaposi's sarcoma. This is a topical treatment.

Side Effects: all localized
Trade Name: Panretin
Skin Effects: itching, rashes, swelling, exfoliative dermatitis, sensations of numbness and prickling

altretamine This medication is used to treat unresponsive ovarian cancer.

Side Effects: nausea, vomiting, anemia, numbness of the extremities
Trade Name: Hexalen
Skin Effects: alopecia, pruritus, rashes

arsenic trioxide This drug is used to treat leukemia.

Side Effects: hypoxia, abdominal pain, back pain
Trade Name: Trisenox
Skin Effects: dermatitis

azacitidine This drug is used to treat leukemia and some types of anemia. It is given subcutaneously.

Side Effects: constipation, fatigue, diarrhea, nausea, anemia, neutropenia, thrombocytopenia, fever, erythema at the injection site
Trade Name: Vidaza
Skin Effects: ecchymosis

methylaminolevulinate This drug is used for the treatment of actinic keratoses, and this medication is used topically.

Side Effects: localized
Trade Name: Metvix
Skin Effects: burning, contact sensitization, erythema, irritation, itching, pain in the area of the application

oxaliplatin This drug is used to treat cancer of the rectum and colon.

Side Effects: fatigue, diarrhea, nausea, vomiting, anemia, neurotoxicity
Trade Name: Eloxatin
Skin Effects: none noted

■ IMPLICATIONS FOR THE SKIN

While many of the drugs associated with chemotherapy have their own sets of skin effects (see below), chemotherapy is easier on the skin than on the hair. However, as a general rule, chemotherapy will dry out the skin because it interferes with the sweat and oil glands that naturally keep the skin moisturized. For clients who are undergoing chemotherapy, there are some key pieces of advice for keeping the skin moist and healthy while undergoing a difficult time. Keeping the skin moisturized will help

Table 13-1 Tips for Caring for the Skin During Chemotherapy
When cleansing, cleanse lightly. Never pull or scrub.
Use an antimicrobial soap.
Moisturize the skin several times a day, especially areas that ordinarily are prone to drying.
Wear rubber gloves when doing household chores.
Wear a sunscreen with at least SPF 15.
Wear lip balm to prevent chapping and cracking of the lips.

Other Cancer Treatment Modalities

RADIATION

Radiation therapy uses high-energy particles or waves, such as x-rays, gamma rays, electrons, or protons to destroy or damage cancer cells. Radiation therapy is one of the most common treatments for cancer. It is often part of the main treatment for some types of cancer, such as cancers of the head and neck, bladder, lung, and Hodgkin's disease. Many other cancers are also treated with radiation therapy. Thousands of people become free of cancer after receiving radiation treatments, either alone or combined with other treatments such as surgery or chemotherapy.

Radiation therapy uses special equipment to deliver high doses of radiation to cancerous cells, killing or damaging them so they cannot grow or spread. It works by breaking a strand of the DNA molecule inside the cancer cell, which prevents the cell from growing and dividing. Although some normal cells may be affected by radiation, most recover fully from the effects of the treatment. Unlike chemotherapy, which exposes the entire body to cancer-fighting chemicals, radiation therapy is a local treatment. It affects only the part of the body being treated.

SURGERY

Surgery is the oldest form of treatment for cancer. It also has an important role in diagnosing and staging (finding the extent) of cancer. Advances in surgical techniques have allowed surgeons to successfully operate on a growing number of patients. Today, more limited (less invasive) operations are often done to remove tumors while preserving as much normal function as possible.

Surgery offers the greatest chance for cure for many types of cancer, especially those that have not yet spread to other parts of the body. Most people with cancer will have some type of surgery.

prevent drying and cracking that could become an infection. Because chemotherapy suppresses the immune system, this is very important.

Conclusion

Cancer can be a devastating disease for those who have it. None of the treatment modalities are easy, and none are 100 percent successful. For patients who undergo chemotherapy, the list of side effects is staggering. Among the list of potential side effects, certain skin effects exist. Some are normal, and others are of potential harm.

As an aesthetician, you can be helpful to any clients who are or will be undergoing treatment for cancer. You should always advise clients to consult their oncologists when you are uncertain or concerned about the nature of a certain skin effect. In addition, you can be a source of comfort to a patient who is going through a difficult time.

REFERENCES

1. http://www.cancer.org
2. http://www.nlm.nih.gov
3. http://www.rxlist.com
4. http://www.drugs.com
5. Deglin, J. H., & Vallerand, A. H. (2007). *Davis's Drug Guide for Nurses.* Philadelphia, PA: F. A. Davis.
6. Michalun, N. (2001). *Milady's Skin Care and Cosmetic Ingredients Dictionary*. Clifton Park: Thomson Delmar Learning.
7. Spratto, G. R., and Woods, A. L. (2005). *2005 PDR Nurse's Drug Handbook.* Clifton Park: Thomson Delmar Learning.
8. http://www.fda.gov

Bone Reabsorption and Antirheumatics

CHAPTER 14

KEY TERMS

Dowager Hump
Etiology
Gingival Hyperplasia
Hirsutism
Liver Toxicity
Osteoarthritis
Paget's Disease

LEARNING OBJECTIVES

After completing this chapter, you should be able to:

1. Discuss bone reabsorption and why it takes place.
2. Discuss some of the ramifications of bone reabsorption.
3. Discuss rheumatoid disease.
4. Discuss some of the common drugs used for the treatment of rheumatoid disease.

INTRODUCTION

Bones and cartilage that are healthy work together to provide a smooth system of operation for the joints. Healthy cartilage is slippery and allows the bones to glide and function unnoticeably, without pain. But over the course of a lifetime the bones and the associated cartilage undergo wear and tear. For some the use is greater, for example, runners who pound their knees against the pavement wear down the cartilage over a period of time, so the bones do not glide as they once did. This, in turn, causes the pain associated with **osteoarthritis**. As time goes on, the joint may collect debris such as chips of bone or cartilage, and the movement may become limited. The good news is that osteoarthritis is a localized condition. Other factors that may contribute to osteoarthritis include obesity and joint injuries.

osteoarthritis
joint condition characterized by inflammation of weight-bearing joints

dowager hump
a bump that forms along the spine occurring due to slow bone loss over time. This most commonly occurs in the elderly.

Rheumatoid arthritis, on the other hand, can affect not only the joints but the internal organs as well. It is considered an autoimmune disease. The immune system protects the body from bacteria, toxins, and harmful substances. The way that this occurs is complex and beyond the scope of this text. But, when the immune system malfunctions (excessive or insufficient performance), certain diseases can occur. It is almost as if the body is "allergic" to itself, attacking normal tissues. The term "autoimmune disease" refers to a varied group of serious, chronic illnesses that involve almost every human organ system. In all of these diseases, the underlying problem is similar—the body's immune system becomes misdirected, attacking the very organs it was designed to protect.

Rheumatoid arthritis is chronic but will typically have times of disease flare and disease remission. During a flare the joints, as well as the tissues around the joints, will be inflamed and sore. If the disease has progressed to a systemic state, the involved organs will also be inflamed. During this time, the patient will be lethargic, and the joints and muscles will be painful and ache. The patient may also be inactive due to the pain. Remissions can occur without reason and last weeks or even years. During times of remission, the patient will feel good, typically without pain.

Another bone disease is osteoporosis. Osteoporosis occurs in both men and women, but it is more common in postmenopausal women when significant bone absorption is likely to occur. Bones that were once strong become porous and brittle. In the spine, the vertebrae begin to compress, and the torso becomes shorter. The appearance of a **dowager hump** becomes more pronounced with time. Certain women are more at risk than others. Those at high risk are Caucasian and Asian women of slight build.

Table 14-1 Autoimmune Diseases

Disease Name	Nature of the Problem
Hashimoto's Disease	Chronic inflammation of the thyroid gland that results in hypothyroidism
Pernicious Anemia	Lack of an intrinsic factor needed to absorb Vitamin B12
Addison's Disease	Hormone deficiency of the adrenal glands
Type I Diabetes	Too little insulin secreted by the pancreas
Rheumatoid Arthritis	Inflammation of the joints and tissue, possibly the organs
Systemic Lupus Erythematosus	Chronic inflammatory disorder that affects the skin, joints, kidneys, and other organs
Dermatomyositis	Inflammation of the skin and muscles
Sjögren's Syndrome	Associated with rheumatic disorders; dry mouth and mucous membranes, decrease in tears
Multiple Sclerosis	Affects the nerves and spinal cord
Myasthenia Gravis	Weakness of voluntary muscle groups
Reiter's Syndrome	Combinations of symptoms, including inflammation of the urethra and joints. Conjunctivitis and lesions of the skin and mucous membranes
Graves' Disease	Overactivity of the thyroid gland
Scleroderma	Chronic disease that is exhibited by systemic sclerosis of the skin
Asthma	Overstimulation of the bronchial tree caused by various stimulants
Fibromyalgia	Chronic pain in the joints and muscles

OSTEOPOROSIS

The treatment of osteoporosis is twofold, first to reduce the pain and second to prevent bone absorption. Typically, the treatment for osteoporosis is focused on a set of dual medications as well as exercise and healthy living. Bone reabsorption medications are usually focused on postmenopausal women.

It is estimated that as many as 70 million Americans suffer from either osteoarthritis or rheumatoid arthritis.

Table 14-2 Risk Factors for Osteoporosis

Influences for Osteoporosis	How Osteoporosis Will Develop
Gender	Postmenopausal women are at the greatest risk
Age	Bones get thinner with age. As aging progresses osteoporosis is more likely
Body Size	Slight sized women are at greater risk
Ethnicity	Caucasians and Asians are at greater risk
Family History	Those individuals with parents who developed osteoporosis may be more likely to develop the disease themselves
Sex Hormones	Absence of periods or low estrogen will influence the development of osteoporosis
Anorexia	Malnourished individuals are at greater risk
Calcium and Vitamin D Intake	Poor bone growth is related to less calcium and vitamin D
Medication Use	Corticosteroids and anticonvulsants can inhibit bone density
Exercise	Lack of exercise will cause the bones to be less dense
Cigarette Smoking	Increases bone loss
Alcohol	Increases bone loss

Biphosphonates

These medications inhibit bone loss in postmenopausal women.

alendronate This medication is used for the treatment of bone loss in postmenopausal women and the treatment of osteoporosis.

Side Effects: stomach pain, constipation, diarrhea, gas, bloating or fullness in the stomach, change in ability to taste food, pain in the muscles or joints, headache, heartburn, upset stomach, vomiting
Trade Name: Fosamax
Skin Effects: rash, photosensitivity, itching, hives, swelling, erythema

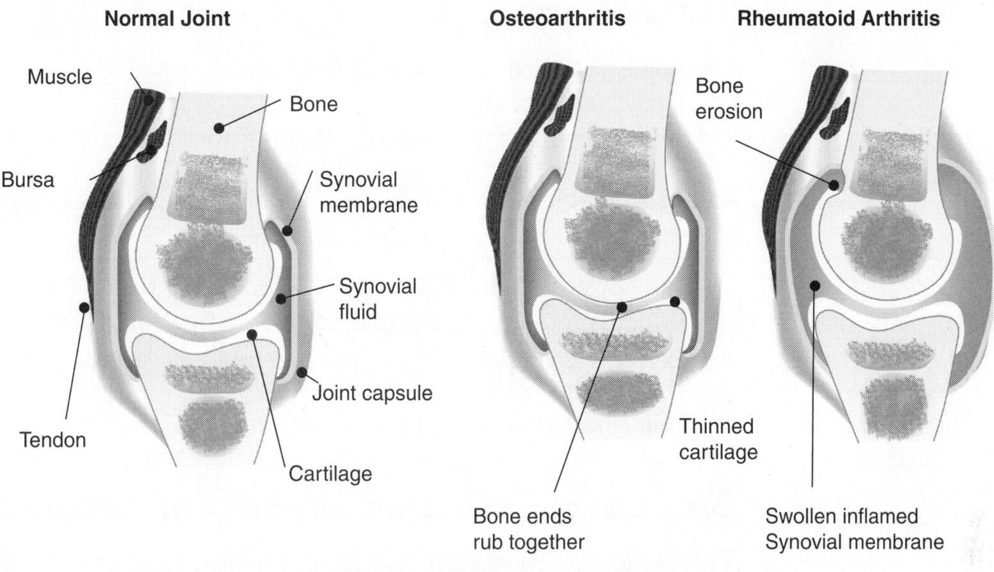

Figure 14-1 Illustration of a normal joint and rheumatoid and osteoarthritis joints

etidronate This medication is used to treat **Paget's disease**; it is also used as a preventative treatment for those undergoing total hip replacements or those with spinal cord injuries.

> **Paget's disease**
> condition affecting the elderly characterized by inflammation of the bones

Side Effects: diarrhea, nausea, bone pain and tenderness
Trade Name: Didronel
Skin Effects: rash

ibandronate This medication is used for the treatment of bone loss in postmenopausal women and the treatment of osteoporosis.

Side Effects: diarrhea, dyspepsia, pain in the extremities
Trade Name: Boniva
Skin Effects: none noted

pamidronate risedronate This medication is used to treat bone loss associated with cancer.

Side Effects: nausea, electrolyte changes, phlebitis at the injection site, muscle stiffness, fever, aches and pains
Trade Name: Aredia
Skin Effects: none noted

tiludronate This medication is used to treat Paget's disease.

Side Effects: side effects are not common
Trade Name: Skelid
Skin Effects: flushing, itching, sweating, rash, and other skin disorders

zoledronic acid This medication is used to treat bone loss associated with cancer.

Side Effects: agitation, anxiety, confusion, trouble sleeping, low blood pressure, abdominal pain, constipation, diarrhea, nausea, vomiting, changes in electrolytes, pain in the bones, fever
Trade Name: Zometa
Skin Effects: rashes, itching

Selective Estrogen Receptor Modulators

This medication works with estrogen receptors to create estrogen effects on the bones.

raloxifene This medication works similar to estrogen to reverse the thinning of bone mass.

Side Effects: hot flashes, muscle pain
Trade Name: Evista
Skin Effects: itching, swelling, skin rash

RHEUMATOID DISEASE

etiology
the study of the cause of a disease

As we have learned, rheumatoid arthritis (RA) is an immune disease, and the **etiology** is unknown. Some scientists have hypothesized that the disease is a result of viruses, bacteria, or fungi, but nothing has been proven. The best scientific guess is that it is genetically inherited or environmentally stimulated. Whatever the cause, treatment after the disease is diagnosed is most important. There are four drug categories for the treatment of RA: DMARDs or disease-modifying antirheumatic drugs, corticosteroids, NSAIDs or nonsteroidal anti-inflammatory drugs, and a group of miscellaneous drugs.

Corticosteroids

Corticosteroids or steroids are powerful drugs that are very helpful to the RA patient as well as to other disease processes associated with inflammation.

Corticosteroids are closely related to the hormones produced within the body, specifically Cortisol, which is manufactured in the adrenal cortex. Steroids reduce the inflammation associated with RA. The table below outlines the steroids used in the treatment of RA, and more information can be found on steroids in Chapter 15.

DMARDs

DMARDs are used to slow the progression of RA. Left untreated, RA can cause deterioration of the joints and eventually irreparable damage. The recent development of DMARDs has allowed those newly diagnosed individuals to be treated before the damage occurs. DMARDs suppress the immune system; therefore, patients taking a medication in this drug category must be educated about the symptoms of infection: chills, fever, sore throat, and cough.

Table 14-3 Corticosteroids Used in the Treatment of Rheumatoid Arthritis

REFER TO CHAPTER 15 FOR MORE INFORMATION

Drug	Trade Name	Use in Rheumatoid Disease
Betamethasone	Celestone	Given orally or by injection to fight inflammation
Cortisone	Cortone Acetate	Given orally or by injection to fight inflammation
Dexamethasone	Decadron	Given orally or by injection to fight inflammation
Hydrocortisone	Cortef, Hydrocortone, Solu-Cortef	Given orally or by injection to fight inflammation
Methylprednisolone	Depo-Medrol, Solu-Medrol	Given orally or by injection to fight inflammation
Prednisolone	Prelone	Given orally or by injection to fight inflammation
Prednisone	Deltasone, Meticorten, Orasone	Given orally or by injection to fight inflammation
Triamcinolone	Kenalog	Given orally or by injection to fight inflammation

anakinra When other DMARDs have failed, this drug can be used alone or in combination with other DMARDs to treat the symptoms of RA. It is given subcutaneously.

Side Effects: pain at the injection site
Trade Name: Kineret
Skin Effects: none noted

etanercept This medication is used for many different types of RA to slow the symptoms of this disease. It is given subcutaneously.

Side Effects: headache, inflammation of the nose, upper respiratory tract infections, pain at the injection site
Trade Name: Enbrel
Skin Effects: none noted

hydroxychloroquine This medication is used frequently to treat the symptoms of autoimmune diseases, including RA.

Side Effects: headache, nausea, vomiting
Trade Name: Plaquenil
Skin Effects: bleaching of the hair, alopecia, hyperpigmentation, photosensitivity, Stevens-Johnson syndrome

infliximab This medication is used for the treatment of RA when the disease is in an active state.

Side Effects: fatigue, headache, upper respiratory tract infections, stomach pain, nausea, vomiting
Trade Name: Remicade
Skin Effects: acne, alopecia, dry skin, ecchymosis, eczema, erythema, flushing, hematoma, increased sweating, hot flashes, itching, hives, rash

leflunomide This medication is used in the treatment of RA.

Side Effects: headache, diarrhea, nausea
Trade Name: Arava
Skin Effects: alopecia, rash, dry skin, eczema, itching

methotrexate This medication is used to treat severe RA.

liver toxicity
abnormal liver functioning sometimes due to drug overdose or hypersensitivity

Side Effects: anorexia, **liver toxicity**, nausea, stomatitis, vomiting, anemia, leukopenia, thrombocytopenia, nephropathy
Trade Names: amethopterin, Folex, Folex PFS, Rheumatrex, Trexall
Skin Effects: alopecia, painful plaque erosions, photosensitivity, itching, rashes, hives, skin ulcers

NSAIDs

Some of the most common drugs consumed by Americans are NSAIDs. They are used to treat a wide variety of ailments, but their most common usage is as a pain reliever. Some of the more common NSAIDs are available in lower dosage OTC versions (ibuprofen, naproxen), but most require a doctor's prescription. More information can be found on NSAIDs in Chapter 17.

Table 14-4 NSAIDs Used in the Treatment of Rheumatoid Arthritis

REFER TO CHAPTER 17 FOR MORE INFORMATION.

Drug	Trade Name	Use in Rheumatoid Disease
Celecoxib	Celebrex	Relief of pain, signs and symptoms of the disease
Flurbiprofen	Ansaid	Relief of pain, signs and symptoms of the disease
Ibuprofen	See Chapter 17	Relief of pain, signs and symptoms of the disease
Indomethacin	Indocin, Indocin IV, Indocin SR	Relief of pain, signs and symptoms of the disease
Ketoprofen	Actron, Orudis, Oruvail	Relief of pain, signs and symptoms of the disease
Nabumetone	Relafen	Relief of pain, signs and symptoms of the disease
Oxaprozin	Daypro	Relief of pain, signs and symptoms of the disease
Piroxicam	Feldene	Relief of pain, signs and symptoms of the disease
Sulindac	Clinoril	Relief of pain, signs and symptoms of the disease
Tolmetin	Tolectin, Tolectin DS	Relief of pain, signs and symptoms of the disease

Miscellaneous Drugs Used in the Treatment of Rheumatoid Disease

The two drugs found in this category are typically used to treat RA that has not responded to other medications.

cyclosporine This drug is an immunosuppressant used in the treatment of RA.

Side Effects: tremor, increased blood pressure, diarrhea, liver toxicity, nausea, vomiting, kidney toxicity, **gingival hyperplasia**, hypersensitivity, infections
Trade Names: Neoral, Sandimmune
Skin Effects: **hirsutism,** acne

gingival hyperplasia
overgrowth of the gums

hirsutism
condition characterized by excessive hair growth in unusual places

sulfasalazine This drug is typically used for the treatment of inflammatory bowel disease, but is also effective in the treatment of RA that is unresponsive to other medications.

Side Effects: headache, anorexia, nausea, vomiting, diarrhea
Trade Name: Azulfidine EN-tabs
Skin Effects: rashes, exfoliative dermatitis, photosensitivity, yellow discoloration of the skin

Conclusion

Here are the facts: in 1985, 35 million Americans suffered from arthritis; in 2005, 66 million, nearly 1 in 3, Americans suffered with arthritis,[1] making it one of the most prevalent diseases in America. Arthritis causes individuals to lose time at work and over time can lead to limits in daily activity. Since the spa is heavily populated with female clients, it is likely that you will frequently see patients taking these drugs. It will be important for you, the aesthetician, to have an understanding of how these drugs impact the skin whether from photosensitivity, rash, or dry skin. All the skin effects may impact the clinical treatment and the patient's ability to tolerate a home care program.

[1] http://www.arthritis.org

REFERENCES

1. http://www.nlm.nih.gov
2. http://www.rxlist.com
3. http://www.drugs.com
4. http://www.arthritis.org
5. Deglin, J. H., & Vallerand, A. H. (2007). *Davis's Drug Guide for Nurses.* Philadelphia, PA: F. A. Davis.
6. Michalun, N. (2001). *Milady's Skin Care and Cosmetic Ingredients Dictionary.* Clifton Park: Thomson Delmar Learning.
7. Roth-Skidmore, Linda. (1999). *1999 Nursing Drug Reference.* St. Louis, MO: Mosby.
8. Spratto, G. R., & Woods, A. L. (2005). *2005 PDR Nurse's Drug Handbook.* Clifton Park: Thomson Delmar Learning.
9. http://www.fda.gov

CHAPTER 15

Corticosteroids

KEY TERMS

Central Serous Retinopathy
Cushing Symptoms
Dysphonia
Folliculitis
Hypertrichoses
Maceration
Metabolic Alkalosis
Miliaria
Oropharynx
Petechiae

LEARNING OBJECTIVES

After completing this chapter, you should be able to:

1. Discuss the use of corticosteroids.
2. Discuss the hazards of corticosteroids.

INTRODUCTION

Cortisones were first introduced in 1949 for the treatment of rheumatoid arthritis. These drugs worked so well, they were deemed "miracles" by the patients using them. Since that time the use of corticosteroids has broadened to include the treatment of other autoimmune diseases such as lupus. Corticosteroids are now also used to treat asthma, adrenal insufficiency, hepatitis, ulcerative bowel disease, and athletic injuries. Topical conditions can also be treated with cortisone; typically the skin and eyes respond well to cortisone.

Corticosteroids when produced naturally attend to the body's stress, immune responses, inflammation, carbohydrate metabolism, protein catabolism, and the blood electrolyte levels. Unfortunately, the results of corticosteroids also come with a price: side effects. The most common side effect is Cushing's syndrome, or moon face. Other side effects include high blood pressure, low potassium in the blood, high sodium levels in the blood, and a condition called **metabolic alkalosis**. Recent studies show that a condition called **central serous retinopathy** or CSR can occur with the use of topical cortisone, nasal sprays containing cortisone, and eye drops containing cortisone.

metabolic alkalosis
increased alkalines in the body resulting from decreased acids

central serous retinopathy
temporary blindness secondary to retinal detachment

dysphonia
hoarseness

oropharynx
the area between the soft palate and upper area of the epiglottis

Corticosteroids, Oral Inhalation

Inhaled corticosteroids are used in the treatment of asthma and may reduce the need for systemic steroids that are sometimes necessary for the treatment of this disease. It has also been found that inhalation corticosteroids may delay the lung damage associated with asthma.

beclomethasone

Side Effects: headache, **dysphonia**, hoarseness, fungal infections in the **oropharynx,** flu-like syndrome
Trade Name: QVAR
Skin Effects: none noted

budesonide

Side Effects: headache, dysphonia, hoarseness, fungal infections in the oropharynx, flu-like syndrome
Trade Name: Pulmicort
Skin Effects: none noted

flunisolide

Side Effects: headache, dysphonia, hoarseness, fungal infections in the oropharynx, flu-like syndrome

Trade Name: AeroBid
Skin Effects: none noted

fluticasone

Side Effects: headache, dysphonia, hoarseness, fungal infections in the oropharynx, flu-like syndrome
Trade Name: Flovent
Skin Effects: none noted

triamcinolone

Side Effects: headache, dysphonia, hoarseness, fungal infections in the oropharynx, flu-like syndrome
Trade Names: Azmacort, Azmacort HFA
Skin Effects: none noted

Corticosteroids, Nasal

These medications are used to treat seasonal allergies and chronic problems with the nose such as nasal polyps. While many of the medications are the same as those in the previous section, bear in mind that they are formulated to be used differently and consequently have different trade names.

beclomethasone

Side Effects: dizziness, headache, stomach pain
Trade Names: Beconase, Beconase AQ, Vancenase, Vancenase AQ 84 mcg
Skin Effects: none noted

budesonide

Side Effects: nasal bleeding, dizziness, headache, stomach pain
Trade Names: Rhinocort, Rhinocort Aqua
Skin Effects: none noted

flunisolide

Side Effects: loss of taste, dizziness, headache, stomach pain
Trade Name: Nasalide
Skin Effects: none noted

fluticasone

Side Effects: dizziness, headache, stomach pain
Trade Name: Flonase
Skin Effects: none noted

mometasone

Side Effects: dizziness, headache, stomach pain
Trade Name: Nasonex
Skin Effects: none noted

triamcinolone

Side Effects: dizziness, headache, stomach pain
Trade Names: Nasacort, Nasacort AQ
Skin Effects: none noted

Corticosteroids, Ophthalmic

This group of corticosteroids is used to treat eye inflammations that may be the result of infections, injury, surgery, or other problems.

dexamethasone

Side Effects: local burning, stinging, irritation, itching, redness, blurred vision, or sensitivity to light
Trade Names: AK-Dex, Decadron Ocumeter, Maxidex
Skin Effects: none noted

fluorometholone

Side Effects: local burning, stinging, irritation, itching, redness, blurred vision, or sensitivity to light
Trade Name: none cited
Skin Effects: none noted

loteprednol

Side Effects: local burning, stinging, irritation, itching, redness, blurred vision, or sensitivity to light
Trade Names: Alrex, Lotemax
Skin Effects: none noted

medrysone

Side Effects: local burning, stinging, irritation, itching, redness, blurred vision, or sensitivity to light
Trade Name: HMS
Skin Effects: none noted

prednisolone

Side Effects: local burning, stinging, irritation, itching, redness, blurred vision, or sensitivity to light

Trade Names: AK-Pred, Econopred, Econopred Plus, Inflamase Forte, Inflamase Mild, Pred Forte, Pred Mild
Skin Effects: none noted

rimexolone

Side Effects: local burning, stinging, irritation, itching, redness, blurred vision, or sensitivity to light
Trade Name: Vexol
Skin Effects: none noted

Corticosteroids, Systemic (Short Acting)

Short acting corticosteroids are used in the treatment of adrenocortical insufficiency; other uses are limited.

cortisone

Cushing Symptoms
relating to Cushing's Disease. Symptoms are: protein loss, adiposity, fatigue and weakness, osteoporosis, amenorrhea, impotence, bruising, swelling, hair growth, diabetes, skin discoloration, changes in skin tugor and striae.

petechiae
red spots on the skin; hemorrhagic spots

Side Effects: depression, euphoria, high blood pressure, anorexia, nausea, muscle wasting, osteoporosis, **Cushing Symptoms** (moon face, buffalo hump)
Trade Name: Cortone Acetate
Skin Effects: acne, delayed wound healing, ecchymoses, fragile skin integrity, hirsutism, **petechiae**

hydrocortisone

Side Effects: depression, euphoria, high blood pressure, anorexia, nausea, muscle wasting, osteoporosis, Cushing Symptoms (moon face, buffalo hump)
Trade Names: Cortef, Solu-Cortef
Skin Effects: acne, delayed wound healing, ecchymoses, fragile skin integrity, hirsutism, petechiae

Corticosteroids, Systemic (Intermediate Acting)

Intermediate acting corticosteroids are used to treat a wide variety of chronic diseases, including but not limited to inflammatory diseases, allergies, autoimmune disorders, cancers, and blood problems.

methylprednisolone

Side Effects: depression, euphoria, high blood pressure, anorexia, nausea, muscle wasting, osteoporosis, Cushing Symptoms (moon face, buffalo hump)

Trade Names: Depo-Medrol, Depro-Medrol, Medrol, Solu-Medrol
Skin Effects: acne, delayed wound healing, ecchymoses, fragile skin integrity, hirsutism, petechiae

prednisolone

Side Effects: depression, euphoria, high blood pressure, anorexia, nausea, muscle wasting, osteoporosis, Cushing Symptoms (moon face, buffalo hump)
Trade Names: Delta-Cortef, Orapred, Pediapred, Prelone
Skin Effects: acne, delayed wound healing, ecchymoses, fragile skin integrity, hirsutism, petechiae

prednisone

Side Effects: depression, euphoria, high blood pressure, anorexia, nausea, muscle wasting, osteoporosis, Cushing Symptoms (moon face, buffalo hump)
Trade Names: Deltasone, Meticorten, Orasone
Skin Effects: acne, delayed wound healing, ecchymoses, fragile skin integrity, hirsutism, petechiae

triamcinolone

Side Effects: depression, euphoria, high blood pressure, anorexia, nausea, muscle wasting, osteoporosis, Cushing Symptoms (moon face, buffalo hump)
Trade Names: Aristocort, Kenalog
Skin Effects: acne, delayed wound healing, ecchymoses, fragile skin integrity, hirsutism, petechiae

Corticosteroids (Long Acting)

Long acting corticosteroids are used to treat a wide variety of chronic diseases, including but not limited to inflammatory diseases, allergies, autoimmune disorders, cancers, and blood problems.

betamethasone

Side Effects: depression, euphoria, high blood pressure, anorexia, nausea, muscle wasting, osteoporosis, Cushing Symptoms (moon face, buffalo hump)
Trade Name: Celestone
Skin Effects: acne, delayed wound healing, ecchymoses, fragile skin integrity, hirsutism, petechiae

budesonide

Side Effects: depression, euphoria, high blood pressure, anorexia, nausea, muscle wasting, osteoporosis, Cushing Symptoms (moon face, buffalo hump)
Trade Name: Entocort EC
Skin Effects: acne, delayed wound healing, ecchymoses, fragile skin integrity, hirsutism, petechiae

dexamethasone

Side Effects: depression, euphoria, high blood pressure, anorexia, nausea, muscle wasting, osteoporosis, Cushing Symptoms (moon face, buffalo hump)
Trade Name: Decadron
Skin Effects: acne, delayed wound healing, ecchymoses, fragile skin integrity, hirsutism, petechiae

Corticosteroids (Topical)

Topical steroids are used frequently in dermatology and medical skin care. Generally, it is said that the application of this product is for the treatment of allergic and immunologic skin problems. It is also commonly used for the treatment of inflammation of the skin after peels or other treatments.

alclometasone

Side Effects: none noted
Trade Name: Aclovate
Skin Effects: allergic contact dermatitis, skin shrinking, burning, dryness, swelling, **folliculitis**, hypersensitivity, **hypertrichoses,** loss of pigmentation, irritation, **maceration**, **miliaria**, perioral dermatitis, secondary infections, stretch marks. With long time use adrenal suppression can occur.

folliculitis
inflammation of the hair follicle

hypertrichoses
excessive hair growth secondary to endocrine disfunction

maceration
making a solid soft with the use of fluid

miliaria
bacterial condition that blocks the sweat glands

amcinonide

Side Effects: none noted
Trade Name: Cyclocort
Skin Effects: allergic contact dermatitis, skin shrinking, burning, dryness, swelling, folliculitis, hypersensitivity, hypertrichoses, loss of pigmentation, irritation, maceration, miliaria, perioral dermatitis, secondary infections, stretch marks. With long time use adrenal suppression can occur.

betamethasone

Side Effects: none noted
Trade Names: Alphatrex, Diprolene, Diprosone, Maxivate, Occlucort, Valisone
Skin Effects: allergic contact dermatitis, skin shrinking, burning, dryness, swelling, folliculitis, hypersensitivity, hypertrichoses, loss of pigmentation, irritation, maceration, miliaria, perioral dermatitis, secondary infections, stretch marks. With long time use adrenal suppression can occur.

clobetasol

Side Effects: none noted
Trade Name: Temovate
Skin Effects: allergic contact dermatitis, skin shrinking, burning, dryness, swelling, folliculitis, hypersensitivity, hypertrichoses, loss of pigmentation, irritation, maceration, miliaria, perioral dermatitis, secondary infections, stretch marks. With long time use adrenal suppression can occur.

clocortolone

Side Effects: none noted
Trade Name: Cloderm
Skin Effects: allergic contact dermatitis, skin shrinking, burning, dryness, swelling, folliculitis, hypersensitivity, hypertrichoses, loss of pigmentation, irritation, maceration, miliaria, perioral dermatitis, secondary infections, stretch marks. With long time use adrenal suppression can occur.

desonide

Side Effects: none noted
Trade Names: DesOwen, Tridesilon
Skin Effects: allergic contact dermatitis, skin shrinking, burning, dryness, swelling, folliculitis, hypersensitivity, hypertrichoses, loss of pigmentation, irritation, maceration, miliaria, perioral dermatitis, secondary infections, stretch marks. With long time use adrenal suppression can occur.

desoximetasone

Side Effects: none noted
Trade Name: Topicort
Skin Effects: allergic contact dermatitis, skin shrinking, burning, dryness, swelling, folliculitis, hypersensitivity, hypertrichoses, loss

of pigmentation, irritation, maceration, miliaria, perioral dermatitis, secondary infections, stretch marks. With long time use adrenal suppression can occur.

dexamethasone

Side Effects: depression, euphoria, increased blood pressure, anorexia, nausea, adrenal suppression, muscle wasting, osteoporosis, moon face
Trade Names: Decadron, Decaspray
Skin Effects: allergic contact dermatitis, skin shrinking, burning, dryness, swelling, folliculitis, hypersensitivity, hypertrichoses, loss of pigmentation, irritation, maceration, miliaria, perioral dermatitis, secondary infections, stretch marks. With long time use adrenal suppression can occur.

diflorasone

Side Effects: none noted
Trade Names: Florone, Maxiflor, Psorcon
Skin Effects: allergic contact dermatitis, skin shrinking, burning, dryness, swelling, folliculitis, hypersensitivity, hypertrichoses, loss of pigmentation, irritation, maceration, miliaria, perioral dermatitis, secondary infections, stretch marks. With long time use adrenal suppression can occur.

fluocinolone

Side Effects: none noted
Trade Names: Derma-Smoothe/FS, FS Shampoo, Synalar, Synemol
Skin Effects: allergic contact dermatitis, skin shrinking, burning, dryness, swelling, folliculitis, hypersensitivity, hypertrichoses, loss of pigmentation, irritation, maceration, miliaria, perioral dermatitis, secondary infections, stretch marks. With long time use adrenal suppression can occur.

fluocinonide

Side Effects: none noted
Trade Name: Lidex
Skin Effects: allergic contact dermatitis, skin shrinking, burning, dryness, swelling, folliculitis, hypersensitivity, hypertrichoses, loss of pigmentation, irritation, maceration, miliaria, perioral dermatitis, secondary infections, stretch marks. With long time use adrenal suppression can occur.

flurandrenolide

Side Effects: none noted
Trade Name: Cordran
Skin Effects: allergic contact dermatitis, skin shrinking, burning, dryness, swelling, folliculitis, hypersensitivity, hypertrichoses, loss of pigmentation, irritation, maceration, miliaria, perioral dermatitis, secondary infections, stretch marks. With long time use adrenal suppression can occur.

fluticasone

Side Effects: none noted
Trade Name: Cutivate
Skin Effects: allergic contact dermatitis, skin shrinking, burning, dryness, swelling, folliculitis, hypersensitivity, hypertrichoses, loss of pigmentation, irritation, maceration, miliaria, perioral dermatitis, secondary infections, stretch marks. With long time use adrenal suppression can occur.

halcinonide

Side Effects: none noted
Trade Name: Halog
Skin Effects: allergic contact dermatitis, skin shrinking, burning, dryness, swelling, folliculitis, hypersensitivity, hypertrichoses, loss of pigmentation, irritation, maceration, miliaria, perioral dermatitis, secondary infections, stretch marks. With long time use adrenal suppression can occur.

halobetasol

Side Effects: none noted
Trade Name: Ultravate
Skin Effects: allergic contact dermatitis, skin shrinking, burning, dryness, swelling, folliculitis, hypersensitivity, hypertrichoses, loss of pigmentation, irritation, maceration, miliaria, perioral dermatitis, secondary infections, stretch marks. With long time use adrenal suppression can occur.

hydrocortisone

Side Effects: none noted
Trade Names: Alphaderm, Anusol HC, Carmol HC, Cort-Dome, Cortenema, Dermacort, DermiCort, Hytone, LactiCare-HC, Locoid, Nutracort, Orabase-HC, Penecort, Proctocort, Westcort

Skin Effects: allergic contact dermatitis, skin shrinking, burning, dryness, swelling, folliculitis, hypersensitivity, hypertrichoses, loss of pigmentation, irritation, maceration, miliaria, perioral dermatitis, secondary infections, stretch marks. With long time use adrenal suppression can occur.

methylprednisolone

Side Effects: none noted
Trade Name: Medrol
Skin Effects: allergic contact dermatitis, skin shrinking, burning, dryness, swelling, folliculitis, hypersensitivity, hypertrichoses, loss of pigmentation, irritation, maceration, miliaria, perioral dermatitis, secondary infections, stretch marks. With long time use adrenal suppression can occur.

mometasone

Side Effects: none noted
Trade Name: Elocon
Skin Effects: allergic contact dermatitis, skin shrinking, burning, dryness, swelling, folliculitis, hypersensitivity, hypertrichoses, loss of pigmentation, irritation, maceration, miliaria, perioral dermatitis, secondary infections, stretch marks. With long time use adrenal suppression can occur.

prednicarbate

Side Effects: none noted
Trade Name: Dermatop
Skin Effects: allergic contact dermatitis, skin shrinking, burning, dryness, swelling, folliculitis, hypersensitivity, hypertrichoses, loss of pigmentation, irritation, maceration, miliaria, perioral dermatitis, secondary infections, stretch marks. With long time use adrenal suppression can occur.

triamcinolone

Side Effects: none noted
Trade Names: Aristocort, Kenalog
Skin Effects: allergic contact dermatitis, skin shrinking, burning, dryness, swelling, folliculitis, hypersensitivity, hypertrichoses, loss of pigmentation, irritation, maceration, miliaria, perioral dermatitis, secondary infections, stretch marks. With long time use adrenal suppression can occur.

Table 15-1 Topical Corticosteroids in Order of Decreasing Class of Potency

Brand Name	Strength	Generic Name
Ultra Highest Potency		
Diprolene	0.05%	betamethasone dipropionate
Temovate	0.05%	clobetasol propionate
Psorcon ointment	0.05%	diflorasone diacetate
Ultravate	0.05%	halobetasol propionate
High Potency		
Cyclocort	0.1%	amcinonide
Alphatrex ointment, cream, lotion Diprosone ointment, cream, lotion Maxivate ointment, cream, lotion	0.05%	betamethasone dipropionate
Topicort	0.25%	desoximetasone
Florone ointment, cream, lotion Maxiflor ointment, cream	0.05%	diflorasone diacetate
Lidex gel, cream, ointment, lotion	0.05%	fluocinonide
Halog ointment, cream, lotion	0.1% and 0.025%	halcinonide
Elocon ointment	0.1%	mometasonefuroate
Diprolene cream and lotion	0.05%	betamethasone dipropionate
Betatrex ointment	0.1%	betamethasone valerate
Valisone ointment	0.1%	betamethasone valerate
Psorcon	0.05%	diflorasone diacetate
Cutivate ointment	0.005%	fluticasone propionate

Continued

Table 15-1 Topical Corticosteroids in Order of Decreasing Class of Potency–cont'd

Aristicort cream, ointment	0.05%	triamcinolone acetonide
Aristicort A cream	0.05%	triamcinolone acetonide
Kenalog cream	0.05%	triamcinolone acetonide
	Moderate Potency	
Topicort LP cream	0.05%	desoximetasone
Synalar ointment	0.025%	fluocinolone acetonide
Cordran	0.05%, 0.025%	flurandrenolide
Westcort ointment	0.2%	hydrocortisone valerate
Elocon	0.1%	mometasone furoate
Aristicort A ointment	0.1%	triamcinolone acetonide
Aristicort ointment	0.1%	triamcinolone acetonide
Kenalog ointment	0.1%	triamcinolone acetonide
Uticort	0.025%	betamethasone benzoate
Diprosone lotion	0.05%	betamethasone dipropioate
Betatrex cream Beta-Val cream	0.1%	betamethasone valerate
Valisone	0.01%	betamethasone valerate
Synalar cream Synemol cream	0.025%	fluocinolone acetonide
Cutivate cream	0.05%	fluticasone propionate
Cordran SP cream	0.05%	flurandrenolide
Locoid	0.1%	hydrocortisone butyrate
Westcort cream	0.2%	hydrocortisone valerate
Kenalog lotion	0.1%	triamcinolone acetonide

Continued

Low Potency		
Aclovate	0.05%	alclometasone dipropionate
Betatrex lotion Beta-Vallotion Valisone lotion	0.1%	betamethasone valerate
DesOwen Tridesilon cream	0.05%	desonide
Fluonid Solution Synalar	0.01%	fluocinolone acetonide
Aristocort cream Aristocort A cream Kenalog Kenalog H cream Triacet cream	0.1%, 0.025%	triamcinolone acetonide
Dermacort Hytone Nutracort Penecort cream Synacort cream	1%	hydrocortisone
Hytone Synacort cream	2.5%	hydrocortisone
Cetacort lotion	0.25%, 0.5%,1%	hydrocortisone
Texacort lotion	0.1%	hydrocortisone
Nutracort lotion	2.5%	hydrocortisone
Cortaid	0.5%,1 %	hydrocortisone acetate
Orabase HCA Oral Paste	0.5%	hydrocortisone acetate

Conclusion

Cortisone is a powerful medication that is used to treat a variety of medical problems. Those in the skin care industry must be alert to a patient who is taking oral cortisone or, more importantly, using topical cortisones. Topical cortisones, as we now have learned, have serious skin effects that the aesthetician should be aware of. The longer the medication is used topically, the greater the risk for skin effects.

A close review of the intake form is important to ascertain if a patient uses cortisone, especially topically. Patients are often placed on topical steroids by the physician following certain surgical procedures such as CO2 laser. It is vital for the aesthetician to know the skin effects of this medication and to keep her or his eyes open for potential problems. The aesthetician's ability to understand the skin effects and work as a valued member of the team is a great resource for the patient and physician alike.

REFERENCES

1. Deglin, J. H., and Vallerand, A. H. (2007). *Davis's Drug Guide for Nurses.* Philadelphia, PA: F. A. Davis.
2. http://www.nlm.nih.gov
3. http://www.rxlist.com
4. http://www.drugs.com
5. Michalun, N. (2001). *Milady's Skin Care and Cosmetic Ingredients Dictionary.* Clifton Park: Thomson Delmar Learning.
6. Spratto, G. R., and Woods, A. L. (2005). *2005 PDR Nurse's Drug Handbook.* Clifton Park: Thomson Delmar Learning.

Hormones

CHAPTER 16

KEY TERMS

Acute Hypoglycemia
Adrenocortical Insufficiency
Asymptomatic
Atrophy
Blood Lipids
Chloasma
Congenital Adrenogenital Syndrome
Endometriosis
Gynecomastia
Hirsutism
Hypercalcemia
Hyperplasia
Hypogonadism
Libido
Melasma
Metabolism
Myalgia
Oligospermia
Perioral
Precocious Puberty
Priapism
Seborrhea
Vasodilation
Vasopressin
Virilism

LEARNING OBJECTIVES

After completing this chapter, you should be able to:

1. Discuss and describe three different hormones.
2. Discuss why the hypothalamus is important in the endocrine system.
3. Name the two types of hormones secreted in the endocrine system.

INTRODUCTION

Compared to other drugs found in this book, the hormones may seem relatively unimpressive both in terms of the number of drugs available to treat hormone-related problems and the different options offered a patient. However, hormones are among the most important molecules in the body. In fact, these hormones are so critical that an overproduction or an underproduction can have serious if not lethal consequences. While a full discussion of the endocrine system is beyond the scope of this text, it is important to have an understanding of the glands that are involved and the substances they secrete.

The endocrine system is a network of glands that secrete or excrete chemical substances or messengers, called hormones, which are released into the blood. Sometimes these glands are part of a larger organ such as the adrenal gland, which is situated on top of the kidney. Endocrine glands secrete these hormones directly into the bloodstream. The endocrine glands include the following: pituitary gland, parathyroid glands, adrenal glands, pineal gland, thymus glands, and the pancreas. Also included are the gonads, more commonly called ovaries and testes. The hypothalamus is also a major contributor to the endocrine system even though it is typically recognized as a part of the nervous system. The hormones produced by these glands are often called chemical messengers. They may aid in the production of other hormones or be antagonistic and work to stop or slow the production of other hormones. The endocrine system secretes two types of hormones: amino acid based or steroid. Prostaglandins, derived from fatty acid molecules and in plasma membranes of the body's cells, are a third category.

Hormones

metabolism
the body's means of processing food into energy

hypercalcemia
high blood calcium

Hormones regulate growth and development, as well as sexual development, maintain the body's ability to fight stress, and balance nutrients, water, and electrolytes, cellular **metabolism**, and energy. A malfunction in one part of the endocrine system often causes another part to malfunction. Assuming that the body does not malfunction, the endocrine system will function properly into old age. However, when the body does malfunction, a synthetic version of the hormone is necessary to keep the body functioning normal.

calcitonin This is used for the treatment of postmenopausal osteoporosis, **hypercalcemia**. This medication is given subcutaneously.

Side Effects: nausea, vomiting, inflammation, symptoms at the injection site

Trade Name: Miacalcin
Skin Effects: rashes

danazol This medication is used in the treatment of **endometriosis**.

Side Effects: emotional lability, deepening of the voice, swelling, loss of menstruation, changes in weight and breast size
Trade Names: Danocrine
Skin Effects: acne, **hirsutism**, oily skin

darbepoetin This medication treats anemia associated with kidney failure and anemia from chemotherapy. This drug is given intravenously and subcutaneously.

Side Effects: dizziness, fatigue, headache, change in blood pressure (high or low), stomach pain, nausea, vomiting, diarrhea, **myalgia,** fever
Trade Name: Aranesp
Skin Effects: itching

desmopressin This medication is used in the treatment of uncontrollable night time bladder and diabetes insipidus due to a decrease in **vasopressin**, as well as to control bleeding in certain circumstances.

Side Effects: rare side effects
Trade Names: DDAVP, DDAVP Rhinal Tube, DDAVP Rhinyle Drops
Skin Effects: flushing

epoetin This medication is used for the treatment of anemia secondary to other treatments such as for HIV/AIDS or cancer.

Side Effects: increased blood pressure
Trade Names: Epogen, EPO, Procrit
Skin Effects: rashes

estrogens These are used topically and systemically as a means of hormone replacement therapy.

Side Effects: headache, inability to wear contacts, swelling, increased blood pressure, nausea, weight changes, changes in menstruation (in men impotence, testicular atrophy, **gynecomastia**), breast tenderness
Trade Names: Premarin, Cenestin, Enjuvia
Skin Effects: acne, oily skin, hyperpigmentation, hives

estropipate This medication is used systemically as a means of hormone replacement therapy.

endometriosis
disease of the endometrium resulting in loss of tissue

hirsutism
condition characterized by excessive hair growth in unusual places

myalgia
muscle pain

vasopressin
hormone that increases blood pressure

gynecomastia
development of abnormally large breasts in men, which may secrete milk

Side Effects: headache, inability to wear contacts, swelling, increased blood pressure, nausea, weight changes, changes in menstruation (in men impotence, testicular atrophy, gynecomastia), breast tenderness
Trade Names: Ogen, Ortho-Est
Skin Effects: acne, oily skin, hyperpigmentation, hives

adrenocortical insufficiency
suppression of one or more of the 50 plus hormones produced in the adrenal cortex

congenital adrenogenital syndrome
a condition characterized by overproduction of male hormones—occurring at birth. In females, this can result in the presence of male sex organs.

acute hypoglycemia
hypoglycemia with rapid onset. See hypoglycemia.

vasodilation
an increase in the flow capacity of veins

blood lipids
concentration of fat in the blood needed for normal functioning

precocious puberty
early onset of puberty

fludrocortisone This medication is used for the treatment of **adrenocortical insufficiency** due to cortisone treatment or **congenital adrenogenital syndrome**.

Side Effects: rare side effects
Trade Name: Florinef
Skin Effects: none noted

glucagon This medication is used for the management of **acute hypoglycemia**, and it is given intravenously or intramuscularly.

Side Effects: nausea, vomiting
Trade Name: Glucagen
Skin Effects: none noted

goserelin This medication is used for the treatment of prostate cancer, endometriosis, and advanced breast cancer.

Side Effects: headache, **vasodilation**, decreased sexual drive, impotence, increase in the **blood lipids**, increase in bone pain, decrease in bone density, hot flashes
Trade Name: Zoladex
Skin Effects: sweating, rashes

insulins These are used for the treatment of diabetes mellitus and diabetes insipidus.

Side Effects: hypoglycemia
Trade Names: Humulin, Iletin, Novolin, Velosulin
Skin Effects: none noted

leuprolide This medication is used in the treatment of prostate cancer, **precocious puberty**, and endometriosis. This medication is given intravenously or subcutaneously or is implanted.

Side Effects: hot flashes
Trade Names: Lupron, Lupron Depot, Lupron Depot-PED, Lupron Depot-3 Month
Skin Effects: none noted

levothyroxine This medication is used for the decrease or absence of thyroid hormone. Also, it is sometimes used to treat thyroid cancers.

Side Effects: insomnia, irritability, nervousness, changes in heartbeat, fast heartbeat, weight loss
Trade Name: Synthroid
Skin Effects: hair loss (children), increased sweating

liothyronine This medication is used for the decrease or absence of thyroid hormone. Also, it is sometimes used to treat thyroid cancers.

Side Effects: insomnia, irritability, nervousness, changes in heartbeat, fast heartbeat, weight loss
Trade Name: Cytomel
Skin Effects: hair loss (children), increased sweating

liotrix This medication is used for the decrease or absence of thyroid hormone. Also, it is sometimes used to treat thyroid cancers.

Side Effects: insomnia, irritability, nervousness, changes in heartbeat, fast heartbeat, weight loss
Trade Name: Thyrolar
Skin Effects: hair loss (children), increased sweating

medroxyprogesterone This medication is used as a contraceptive (see below). It is also used to decrease endometrial **hyperplasia**, as well as to treat irregular bleeding and renal cancer.

Side Effects: rare side effect
Trade Names: Amen, Cycrin, Depo-Provera, Depo-Sub Q Provera 104, Provera
Skin Effects: melasma, rash

megestrol This medication is used for the palliative treatment of endometrial and breast cancer.

Side Effects: **asymptomatic** adrenal suppression with chronic treatment
Trade Name: Megace
Skin Effects: none noted

nafarelin This medication is used for the management of endometriosis.

Side Effects: changes in mood, headaches, nasal irritation, vaginal dryness, end of menses, changes in fertility, reduction in breast size, decreased libido, hot flashes

hyperplasia
excessive proliferation of normal cell in tissue

asymptomatic
not presenting with any noticeable symptoms

seborrhea
condition characterized by excessive sebaceous secretion

virilism
the presence of male patterned hair growth on women

chloasma
yellow or brown mispigmentation of the skin

melasma
general name for discoloration of the skin

Trade Name: Synarel
Skin Effects: acne, hirsutism, **seborrhea**

nandrolone decanoate This medication is used for the treatment of anemia due to renal insufficiency.

Side Effects: **virilism** in women and prepubertal men
Trade Names: Deca-Durabolin, Hybolin Decanoate
Skin Effects: acne

octreotide This medication is used to treat diarrhea and flushing for patients with endocrine tumors.

Side Effects: rare side effects
Trade Names: Sandostatin, Sandostatin LAR
Skin Effects: flushing

oxytocin This medication is used for the induction of labor.

Side Effects: increased uterine motility, painful contractions
Trade Name: Pitocin
Skin Effects: none noted

progestins This medication is used topically and systemically as a means of hormone replacement therapy.

Side Effects: rare side effects
Trade Names: Crinone, Prochieve, Prometrium
Skin Effects: **chloasma**, **melasma**, rashes

somatrem (recombinant) This medication is used to treat growth failure in children.

Side Effects: rare side effects
Trade Names: Genotropin, Genotropin MiniQuick, Humatrope, Norditropin cartridges, Norditropin NordiFlex, Nutropin, Nutropin AQ, Protropin, Saizen, Serostim
Skin Effects: none noted

somatropin (recombinant) This medication is used to treat growth failure in children.

Side Effects: rare side effects
Trade Names: Genotropin, Humatrope, Norditropin, Nutropin, Nutropin AQ, Nutropin Depot, Saizen, Serostim, Serostim LQ, Tev-Tropin, Zorbtive
Skin Effects: none noted

teriparatide This medication is used for the treatment of osteoporosis.

Side Effects: rare side effects
Trade Name: Forteo
Skin Effects: none noted

testosterone This medication is used for the treatment of **hypogonadism** in androgen-deficient men.

Side Effects: swelling; for women: changes in **libido**, clitoral enlargement, decreased breast size; for men: gynecomastia, impotence, **oligospermia**, **priapism**
Trade Names: Andro, Histerone, Testamone, Testaqua, Testoject, Striant, Andro-Cyp, Andronate, depAndro, Depotest, Depo-Testosterone, Duratest, T-Cypionate, Testa-C, Testred, Testoject-LA, Virilon IM, Andro LA, Andropository, Andryl, Delatest, Delatestryl, Everone, Testone LA, Testrin-PA, Testex, Androderm, AndroGel, Testim
Skin Effects: for men: acne and facial hair

hypogonadism
condition characterized by underdevelopment of the gonads and secondary sexual characteristics

libido
sexual desire

oligospermia
low sperm count

priapism
a prolonged erection without sexual desire

perioral
around the mouth

thyroid This medication is used for the decrease or absence of thyroid hormone. Also, it is sometimes used to treat thyroid cancers.

Side Effects: insomnia, irritability, nervousness, changes in heartbeat, fast heartbeat, weight loss
Trade Name: Armour thyroid
Skin Effects: hair loss (children), increased sweating

triptorelin This medication is used for the palliative treatment of prostate cancer.

Side Effects: pain in the bones and muscles, impotence
Trade Names: Trelstar Depot
Skin Effects: itching

vasopressin This medication is used for diabetes insipidus due to insufficient antidiuretic hormone and is given intramuscularly and intravenously.

Side Effects: rare side effects
Trade Name: Pitressin
Skin Effects: paleness, **perioral** blanching, sweating

CONTRACEPTIVE HORMONES

Drugs used to prevent pregnancy are called contraceptives or, more commonly, birth control pills (BCP). Birth control medications are made up of the hormones estrogen and progesterone. The goal of these medications is to prevent a pregnancy, which is accomplished in a few different ways. Some birth control medications block ovulation, others hinder sperm transport, and others manipulate the fallopian tubes or the endometrium.

Birth control is delivered in a variety of manners, including pills, intravenous methods, topical patches, and slow release systems (such as rings and skin implants). The most effective medication will vary from one individual to the next. Ideally, the medication should control the menstrual cycle with minimal side effects. The types of birth control are determined and named by the doses of progestin and estrogen in each of the active pills. The four dosages are referred to as monophasic, biphasic, triphasic, and progesterone-only pills (POP). Many patients will need to work with their physicians, changing their prescription a few times to find out which is best for them.

Monophasic pills have a constant dose of both estrogen and progestin in each of the hormonally active pills throughout the entire cycle (21 days of ingesting active pills). Several of the brands may be available in differing strengths of estrogen or progesterone, from which the physician can choose according to a woman's individual needs. Biphasic pills typically contain two different progesterone doses. The progesterone dose is increased about halfway through the cycle. Triphasic pills gradually increase the dose of estrogen during the cycle (some pills also increase the progesterone dose). Three different increasing pill doses are contained in each cycle. Progesterone-only pills (POPs), also known as mini-pills, are not used widely in the United States. Less than 1 percent of users of oral contraceptives use them as their only method of birth control. Those who use them include women who are breastfeeding and women who cannot take estrogen.

There are certain drug interactions that are important to know when a client is taking BCP. Among the most important is the decreased efficacy of BCP with certain antibiotics such as penicillin or tetracycline. Because tetracycline is often used in the treatment of acne, the client should be educated about the possible interference with BCP.

It should also be mentioned that BCP can be used for the management of acne. The most common BCP used for this purpose is Ortho Tri-Cyclen. The aesthetician can suggest this option to a client and encourage her to seek the help of a qualified physician. This can be recommended to a client in moderate to severe cases. The client should seek out a patient and willing physician who is empathic to the problems of acne.

estradiol acetate

Side Effects: headache, inability to wear contact lenses, swelling, high blood pressure, nausea, weight changes, changes in menstruation,

Table 16-1 Drugs That Can Interfere with BCP

Drug	Interaction	Possible Result
Penicillin, ampicillin, oral neomycin, tetracycline	Decrease the efficacy of BCP	Pregnancy
Chloramphenicol, dihydroergotamine, mineral oil, sulfonamides, barbiturates	Decrease the efficacy of BCP	Pregnancy
Chronic alcohol use	Decrease the efficacy of BCP	Pregnancy
Carbamazepine (Tegretol), oxcarbazepine (Trileptal)	Decrease the efficacy of BCP	Pregnancy
Systemic corticosteroids, phenylbutazone, phenytoin, topiramate, primidone, bosentan modafinil, rifampin, some protease inhibitor antiretrovials (ritonavir)	Decrease the efficacy of BCP	Pregnancy
Tricyclic antidepressants	Increase the effects of these drugs	Possible toxicity
Some benzodiazepine, beta blockers, caffeine, corticosteroids, cyclosporins, and theophylline	Increase the effects of these drugs	Possible toxicity
Dantrolene (with estrogen only)	Increased risk of hepatic toxicity	Problems associated with liver toxicity
Carbamazepine or phenytoin	Decrease the efficacy of BCP	Pregnancy

Continued

Table 16-1 Drugs That Can Interfere with BCP–cont'd		
Bromocriptine	Changes the levels of this drug	Ineffective
Acetaminophen, temazepan, lorazepam, oxazepam, salicylic acid, morphine	Decreases the levels of these drugs	Less effective
NSAIDs, potassium-sparing diuretics, potassium supplements, ACE inhibitors, angiotensin II receptor antagonists, or heparin	Increases in blood potassium	Changes in cardiac rhythm
St. John's Wort	Decrease the efficacy Irregular menses	Pregnancy
Cola nut, coffee, tea	Increase caffeine levels	Increase side effects of caffeine

atrophy
loss of muscle tissue most often from inactivity

Hormones

gynecomastia, and breast tenderness; in men: testicular **atrophy** and impotence
Trade Name: Femtrace
Skin Effects: oily skin, acne, pigmentation, hives

estradiol cypionate

Side Effects: headache, inability to wear contact lenses, swelling, high blood pressure, nausea, weight changes, changes in menstruation, gynecomastia, and breast tenderness; in men: testicular atrophy and impotence
Trade Names: depGynogen, Depo-Estradiol, Depogen, Dura-Estrin, E-Cypionate, Estragyn LA 5, Estro-Cyp, Estrofem, Estroject LA, Estro-L.A.
Skin Effects: oily skin, acne, pigmentation, hives

estradiol cypionate/medroxyprogesterone acetate

Side Effects: rare side effects

Trade Name: Lunelle
Skin Effects: melasma, rash

estradiol valerate

Side Effects: headache, inability to wear contact lenses, swelling, high blood pressure, nausea, weight changes, changes in menstruation, gynecomastia, and breast tenderness; in men: testicular atrophy and impotence
Trade Name: Delestrogen
Skin Effects: oily skin, acne, pigmentation, hives

estradiol topical emulsion

Side Effects: headache, inability to wear contact lenses, swelling, high blood pressure, nausea, weight changes, changes in menstruation, gynecomastia, and breast tenderness; in men: testicular atrophy and impotence
Trade Name: Estrasorb
Skin Effects: oily skin, acne, pigmentation, hives

estradiol transdermal system

Side Effects: headache, inability to wear contact lenses, swelling, high blood pressure, nausea, weight changes, changes in menstruation, gynecomastia, and breast tenderness; in men: testicular atrophy and impotence
Trade Names: Alora, Climara, Esclim, Estraderm, FemPatch, Menostar, Vivelle
Skin Effects: oily skin, acne, pigmentation, hives

estradiol valginal tablet

Side Effects: headache, inability to wear contact lenses, swelling, high blood pressure, nausea, weight changes, changes in menstruation, gynecomastia, and breast tenderness; in men: testicular atrophy and impotence
Trade Name: Vagifem
Skin Effects: oily skin, acne, pigmentation, hives

estradiol vaginal ring

Side Effects: headache, inability to wear contact lenses, swelling, high blood pressure, nausea, weight changes, changes in menstruation, gynecomastia, and breast tenderness; in men: testicular atrophy and impotence

Trade Names: Femring, Estring
Skin Effects: oily skin, acne, pigmentation, hives

ethinyl estradiol/desogestrel

Side Effects: rare side effects
Trade Names:
Monophasic Trade Names: Desogen, Ortho-Cept
Triphasic Trade Names: Cyclessa, Velivet
Skin Effects: melasma, rash

ethinyl estradiol/drospirenone

Side Effects: rare side effects
Trade Name: Yasmin
Skin Effects: melasma, rash

ethinyl estradiol/ethynodiol

Side Effects: rare side effects
Trade Names: Demulen, Demulen 1/35
Skin Effects: melasma, rash

ethinyl estradiol/etonogestrel

Side Effects: rare side effects
Trade Name: NuvaRing
Skin Effects: melasma, rash

ethinyl estradiol/levonorgestrel

Side Effects: rare side effects
Trade Names: Alesse, Aviane-28, Levlen, Lutera, Nordette
Skin Effects: melasma, rash

ethinyl estradiol/norelgestromin

Side Effects: rare side effects
Trade Name: Ortho Evra
Skin Effects: melasma, rash

ethinyl estradiol /norethindrone

Side Effects: rare side effects
Trade Names:
Monophasic Trade Names: Brevicon, Genora 0.5/35, Genora 1/35, Junel 21 1/20, Junel 21 15/20, Loestrin 21 1.5/30, Loestrin 21 1/20, Microgestin, Modicon N.E.E. 1/35, Nelova

0.5/35E, Nelova 1/35E, Norcept-E1/35, Norethin 1/35E, Norinyl 1+35, Norlestrin 1/50, Norlestrin 2.5/50, Nortrel, Ortho-Novum 1/35, Ovcon 35, Ovcon 50

Biphasic Trade Names: Kariva, Mircette, Nelova 10/11, Ortho-Novum 10/11

Triphasic Trade Names: Aranelle, Necor 7/7/7, Nortrel 7/7/7, Ortho-Novum 7/7/7, Tri-Norinyl

Skin Effects: melasma, rash

ethinyl estradiol/norgestimate

Side Effects: rare side effects
Trade Names: Ortho-Cyclen, Previfem, Sprintec
Skin Effects: melasma, rash

ethinyl estradiol/norgestrel

Side Effects: rare side effects
Trade Names:
Monophasic Trade Names: Cryselle, Lo/Ovral, Ovral
Triphasic Trade Names: Enpresse, Portia, Tri-Levlen, Triphasil
Skin Effects: melasma, rash

levonorgestrel

Side Effects: rare side effects
Trade Names: Mirena, Plan B
Skin Effects: melasma, rash

levonorgestrel/ethinyl estradiol

Side Effects: rare side effects
Trade Name: Preven
Skin Effects: melasma, rash

medroxyprogesterone

Side Effects: rare side effects
Trade Names: Depo-Provera, Depo-subQ, Provera 104
Skin Effects: melasma, rash

mestranol/norethindrone

Side Effects: rare side effects
Trade Names: Genora 1/50, Nelova 1/50M, Norethin 1/50M, Norinyl 1+50, Ortho-Novum 1/50, Yasmin
Skin Effects: melasma, rash

norethindrone

Side Effects: rare side effects
Trade Names: Errin, Ortho Micronor, Camila, Jolivette, Nor-QD
Skin Effects: melasma, rash

norethindrone/ethinyl acetate

Side Effects: rare side effects
Trade Names: Estrostep, Estrostep Fe
Skin Effects: melasma, rash

norgestimate/ethinyl estradiol

Side Effects: rare side effects
Trade Names: Ortho Tri-Cyclen, Ortho Tri-Cyclen Lo
Skin Effects: melasma, rash

norgestrel

Side Effects: rare side effects
Trade Name: Ovrette
Skin Effects: melasma, rash

Conclusion

As we have learned, hormones vary widely and affect the body in many different ways. In most cases a hormone can regulate the production and release of other hormones. An underabundance of a specific hormone can cause a ripple effect with the end result being a sick patient.

While the aesthetician does not need to know all of the glands of the endocrine system or all of the hormones secreted, it is important for the aesthetician to know and understand that hormones affect the skin, hair, and nails. Conditions such as acne, melasma, dry skin, and hair loss can be the result of hormone fluctuations from life cycle changes. If your patient is on a particular hormone, understanding that hormone deficiency and the side effects associated therein will be valuable for the clinician and the patient alike.

REFERENCES

1. http://www.mayoclinic.com/health/hormone-therapy/WO00046
2. http://www.merck.com
3. Deglin, J. H., & Vallerand, A. H. (2007). *Davis's Drug Guide for Nurses.* Philadelphia, PA: F. A. Davis.

Drugs Used to Treat Pain

CHAPTER 17

KEY TERMS

Ankylosing Spondylitis
Apnea
Conjunctivitis
Cyanosis
Diplopia
Dysphoria
Euphoria
Hemoptysis
Narcotic
Nasopharyngitis
Opioid Detoxification
Paresthesia
Positive Stool Guaiac
Spasticity
Stevens-Johnson Syndrome
Supraspinatus
Syncope
Tinnitus
Toxic Epidermal Necrolysis

LEARNING OBJECTIVES

After completing this chapter, you should be able to:

1. Understand the difference between narcotic analgesics and non-narcotic analgesics.
2. Identify some of the common side effects associated with nonsteroidal anti-inflammatory drugs.
3. Know the common responses the skin has to these drugs.

INTRODUCTION

The description of pain is divided into two categories, either chronic or acute. Chronic pain is that pain associated with everyday causes, for example, arthritis, while acute pain is associated with injury or surgery. Whether the pain is chronic or acute its relief is important to allow a patient to return to as normal a life as possible. Often the relief is associated with a medication that manages and lessens the pain.

Pain medications can reduce inflammation and pain when taken properly. Although pain medications cannot stop the effects of aging and wear and tear on the body, they can help control pain. Likewise, pain medications do not remedy the underlying cause, but they do make certain conditions more manageable.

Pain medications also are associated with a certain amount of risk. Many pain medications are addictive and often abused. Great concern and restraint must be executed when taking pain medications.

SKIN IMPLICATIONS FOR PAIN MEDICATIONS

It is important for the aesthetician to know that certain drugs have skin effects that may appear on patients taking these drugs. As the aesthetician, you should take a complete health history during the consultative process, which includes a detailed list of all medications that the client is taking.

With pain medications, the primary concern involves rashes, which are usually associated with allergic reactions. If you suspect that your client is experiencing an allergic reaction, refer him or her to a physician. Allergic reactions can sometimes be severe, and the treatments are outside the scope of an aesthetician's abilities.

It is possible that clients may complain of skin conditions that are not known to have been caused by their medications. For instance, pruritus and erythema are common skin effects of many medications. These symptoms while not clearly allergic in nature could be a sign of hypersensitivity and the patient should be referred to the physician.

TYPES OF PAIN

There are four pain classifications that we will discuss: acute pain, chronic nonmalignant pain, chronic malignant pain, and headaches. Headaches are the most common source of pain and can be considered a separate class since they can be both acute and chronic, as well as malignant or nonmalignant.

Acute pain is sudden onset pain, most often associated with trauma. This trauma is usually caused by mechanical means or accidents that result in torn ligaments, broken bones, bruises, and cuts. The degree to which pain management is necessary is related to the severity of the trauma. A cut may require only an over-the-counter (OTC) remedy, whereas the incision associated with a surgery may require something stronger.

Chronic nonmalignant pain is associated with progressive diseases, such as arthritis. OTC medications for pain usually are effective for this type of pain. However, more recently, pharmaceutical companies have been developing newer drugs that manage the pain without the tranquilizing effects of narcotic pain medications.

Chronic malignant pain is associated with progressive diseases that are often fatal, such as cancer, Parkinson's disease, or multiple sclerosis. These illnesses are often painful and require a stronger pain killer for extended periods of time. As mentioned, headaches are the most common cause of pain. They are classified into three types: muscle contraction headaches, migraine headaches, and sinus headaches.

The first type of headache is also the most common: muscle contraction headaches. They are the product of prolonged and continuous tightening of the muscles in the upper back, neck, or scalp. The pain associated with these headaches is often described as throbbing or tightness in the back or sides of the head. Often, stress or posture is the culprit for these headaches. Acute muscle contraction headaches respond well to OTC analgesics, but sometimes require physical therapy or massage to remedy them in the long term.

The second type of headache is called a migraine. Migraines are caused by a dilation of blood vessels in the head. Women are twice as likely to suffer from migraine headaches as are men. They are often extremely painful and recurrent. OTC pain relief associated with migraines varies from one individual to the next. Therefore, prescription medications specifically intended for treating or preventing migraines often are necessary.

Finally, sinus headaches are caused by an infection or blockage within the sinus cavities of the head. Sinus headache pain is often limited to the face and nose, as well as areas surrounding the major cavities. OTC remedies with decongestive additives are often effective for treating sinus headaches.

NARCOTIC ANALGESICS

Narcotic analgesics are a class of pain medications that are considered to be habit-forming. They act on the central nervous system to control and relieve pain. Narcotics are prescription medications. In children and

narcotic
a drug that is both physically and psychologically addictive, but has medicinal benefits

older adults the use of narcotic agents can depress the respiratory function. The use of narcotics in pregnant women has not been studied. The results of any impact of narcotics on the unborn fetus have been studied only in animals. Narcotics should be used with care in pregnant and breast-feeding women.

There are certain drugs that should not be taken in conjunction with narcotics. Normally a physician would make this determination and evaluate the patient accordingly. There are certain health conditions that might prohibit the use of a narcotic agent. These might include alcohol abuse and drug addiction. Other health problems might cause the physician to pause and reevaluate. These conditions include emotional problems, head injuries, brain diseases, lung diseases, urinary problems, gallbladder problems, intestinal problems, and heart disease. Other problems that might preclude the use of narcotic analgesics are kidney disease, liver disease, thyroid problems, and, most especially, convulsions.

buprenorphine relief of moderate to severe pain

Side Effects: nausea, dizziness/vertigo, sweating, vomiting, headache, constipation, **cyanosis, diplopia**, visual abnormalities, urinary retention, dreaming, warmth, cold/chills, **tinnitus, conjunctivitis,** psychosis, lack of muscle coordination, physical and psychological dependence
Trade Names: Buprenex, Subutex
Skin Effects: pruritus, rash, flushing, urticaria

cyanosis
bluish coloring of the skin resulting from reduced levels of hemoglobin in the blood

diplopia
seeing double

tinnitus
ringing in the ears

conjunctivitis
inflammation of the mucous membranes of the eyes and eyelids

dysphoria
feelings of depression, discomfort, or unhappiness with no known cause

butorphanol relief of moderate to severe pain

Side Effects: confusion, **dysphoria**, hallucinations, sedation, nausea, vomiting, urinary retention, physical and psychological dependence
Trade Names: Stadol, Stadol NS
Skin Effects: sweating, clammy skin

codeine for the treatment of mild to moderately severe pain

Side Effects: lightheadedness, dizziness, sedation, shortness of breath, nausea, vomiting, euphoria, dysphoria, constipation, abdominal pain, physical and psychological dependence
Trade Names: Tylenol with Codeine, Acetaminophen with Codeine, Butalbital, Fiorinal, Guaifenesin
Skin Effects: pruritus

fentanyl citrate for the treatment of persistent pain to chronic severe pain

Side Effects: loss of strength, headache, nausea, vomiting, constipation, dizziness, sleepiness, confusion, anxiety, difficulty walking,

dry mouth, nervousness, vasodilation, hallucinations, insomnia, difficulty thinking straight, vertigo, dyspnea, abnormal vision, physical and psychological dependence
Trade Name: Actiq
Skin Effects: pruritus, rash, sweating

fentanyl transdermal system for the treatment of moderate to severe pain that requires around the clock attention

Side Effects: abdominal pain, headache, fatigue, back pain, fever, flu-like symptoms, rigor, arrhythmia, chest pain, nausea, vomiting, constipation, dry mouth, anorexia, diarrhea, dyspepsia, flatulence, loss of strength, insomnia, confusion, sleepiness, nervousness, hallucination, anxiety, depression, **euphoria,** tremors and abnormal coordination, abnormal speech, abnormal walking, bad dreams, agitation, **paresthesia,** amnesia, **syncope,** paranoid behaviors, dyspnea, hypoventilation, **apnea, hemoptysis,** pharyngitis, hiccups, bronchitis, rhinitis, sinusitis, upper respiratory tract infections, urinary tract infections, changes in urination, physical and psychological dependence
Trade Name: Duragesic
Skin Effects: sweating, pruritus, rash at the application site, erythema, papules, itching, edema

hydrocodone treatment of moderate to severe pain

Side Effects: drowsiness, clouded judgment, lethargy, anxiety and fear, dysphoria, psychic dependence, mood changes, constipation, ureteral spasm, spasm of sphincters, urinary retention, respiratory depression, possible permanent hearing loss, physical and psychological dependence
Trade Names: Lortab, Vicodin, Zydone
Skin Effects: rashes, pruritus

hydromorphone 24 hour relief of moderate to severe pain

Common Side Effects: confusion, hypotension, constipation, dry mouth, nausea, vomiting, physical and psychological dependence
Trade Name: Dilaudid
Skin Effects: flushing, sweating

meperidine hydrochloride used for the treatment of acute severe pain

Side Effects: dizziness, lightheadedness, drowsiness, mood changes, upset stomach, vomiting, constipation, difficulty urinating, physical and psychological dependence

euphoria
temporary state of excitement and happiness

paresthesia
sensation of numbness and prickling; often called "pins and needles"

syncope
a momentary loss of blood flow to the brain resulting in unconsciousness

apnea
temporary ceasing of normal breathing function; often happening while sleeping

hemoptysis
coughing up blood

Trade Name: Demerol
Skin Effects: sweating, rash

opioid detoxification to reduce the toxic properties of addictive drugs

methadone management of severe pain and **opioid detoxification**

Side Effects: confusion, sedation, dizziness, hallucinations, hypotension, nausea, vomiting, constipation, physical and psychological dependence
Trade Name: Methadose
Skin Effects: flushing, sweating

morphine used for severe pain

Side Effects: drowsiness, changes in mood, respiratory depression, decreased gastrointestinal movement, nausea, vomiting, alterations of the endocrine and autonomic central nervous system, physical and psychological dependence
Trade Name: known as morphine
Skin Effects: dry skin, urticaria

nalbuphine relief of moderate to severe pain

Side Effects: dizziness, headache, sedation, hallucinations, dry mouth, nausea, vomiting, constipation, physical and psychological dependence
Trade Name: Nubain
Skin Effects: sweating and clammy skin

oxycodone used for the management of severe pain with around the clock needs

Side Effects: anorexia, nervousness, insomnia, fever, confusion, diarrhea, abdominal pain, dyspepsia, anxiety, euphoria, dyspnea, postural hypotension, chills, twitching, gastritis, abnormal dreams, hiccups, physical and psychological dependence
Trade Names: Combunox, OxyContin, Percocet, Percodan, Endocet
Skin Effects: rashes, dry skin, exfoliative dermatitis, urticaria

oxymorphone relief of moderate to severe pain

Common Side Effects: confusion, sedation, dizziness, blurred vision, nausea, vomiting, constipation, physical and psychological dependence
Trade Name: Numorphan
Skin Effects: flushing, sweating

propoxyphene for use in the resolution of mild to moderate pain

Side Effects: dizziness, sedation, nausea, vomiting, constipation, abdominal pain, lightheadedness, headaches, weakness, euphoria,

dysphoria, hallucinations and visual disturbances, physical and psychological dependence
Trade Name: Darvon
Skin Effects: skin rashes

NONSTEROIDAL ANTI-INFLAMMATORY DRUGS

Some of the most common drugs consumed by Americans are nonsteroidal anti-inflammatory drugs (NSAIDs). They are used to treat a wide variety of ailments, but their most common usage is as a pain reliever. Some of the more common NSAIDs are available in lower dosage OTC versions (Ibuprofen, Naproxen), but most require a doctors prescription.

NSAIDs also are associated with some consequential side effects, some of which can be life threatening when used regularly over extended periods of time. One such example is Celebrex. Celebrex was originally approved by the FDA to treat rheumatoid arthritis. Later it was pulled from the shelves after it was shown that it may cause an increased risk of serious cardiovascular thrombotic events, myocardial infarction, and stroke, which can be fatal. All NSAIDs may have a similar risk. This risk may increase with duration of use. Patients with cardiovascular disease or risk factors for cardiovascular disease may be at greater risk; heart attack, stroke, chest pain, shortness of breath, weakness, and slurring of speech are common with these drugs

celecoxib a nonsteroidal anti-inflammatory drug used for the management of pain in osteoarthritis, rheumatoid arthritis, **ankylosing spondylitis**

ankylosing spondylitis stiffening of the vertebrae in the spine resulting in loss of movement

Side Effects: abdominal pain, diarrhea, dyspepsia, flatulence, nausea, heart attack, stroke, chest pain, shortness of breath, weakness, slurring of speech, edema, weight gain, back pain, flu-like symptoms, dizziness, headache, insomnia, pharyngitis, rhinitis, sinusitis, upper respiratory tract infections
Trade Name: Celebrex
Skin Effects: can cause serious skin side effects including exfoliative dermatitis, Stevens-Johnson syndrome, toxic epidermal necrolysis; also, simple problems such as rash, blisters, and itching

diclofenac for treatment of menstrual cramps, mild to moderate pain associated with osteoarthritis and rheumatoid arthritis

Side Effects: abdominal pain, constipation, diarrhea, dyspepsia, flatulence, GI bleeding and perforation, heartburn, nausea, GI ulcers,

vomiting, abnormal renal function, anemia, dizziness, edema, elevated liver enzymes, headaches, increased bleeding time, tinnitus
Trade Names: Cataflam, Voltaren
Skin Effects: pruritus, rash

diflunisal for the treatment of mild to moderate pain, the pain associated with osteoarthritis and rheumatoid arthritis

Side Effects: heart attack, stroke, high blood pressure, heart failure, kidney failure, GI bleeding and ulcers, anemia, liver failure, asthma attacks, stomach pain, constipation, diarrhea, flatulence, heartburn, nausea, vomiting, dizziness
Trade Name: Dolobid
Skin Effects: skin rashes or blisters, fever; rarely: erythema multiforme, exfoliative dermatitis, **Stevens-Johnson syndrome, toxic epidermal necrolysis,** urticaria, pruritus, sweating, dry mucous membranes, stomatitis, photosensitivity

Stevens-Johnson syndrome
A systemic form of erythema multiforme, with lesions of the mucous membranes and a severe rash

toxic epidermal necrolysis
see epidermal necrolysis

nasopharyngitis
inflammation of nasopharynix

etodolac used to treat the pain and inflammation associated with rheumatoid arthritis and osteoarthritis; occasionally used to treat ankylosing spondylitis, tendonitis, bursitis, painful shoulder, gout

Side Effects: stomach pain, diarrhea, gas or bloating, upset stomach, weakness, dizziness, depression, chills, nervousness, constipation, vomiting, painful or frequent urination, black and tarry stools, red blood in stools, bloody vomit, vomiting material that looks like coffee grounds, blurred vision, swelling of the hands, feet, ankles, or lower legs, unexplained weight gain, difficulty breathing or swallowing, yellowing of the skin or eyes, ringing in the ears
Trade Name: Lodine
Skin Effects: pale skin, rash, itching, hives

fenoprofen for the pain associated with rheumatoid arthritis; for acute flare-ups and exacerbations associated with the management of rheumatoid arthritis

Side Effects: greatest number of side effects are gastrointestinal in nature, including nausea, constipation, vomiting, abdominal pain, diarrhea; other side effects include dizziness, confusion, tinnitus, blurred vision, palpitations, nervousness, asthenia, peripheral edema, dyspnea, fatigue, upper respiratory infections, **nasopharyngitis**
Trade Name: Nalfon
Skin Effects: increased sweating, pruritus, rash

flurbiprofen for the treatment of arthritis, including the pain, stiffness, tenderness, and swelling associated with this disease

Side Effects: headache, dizziness, nervousness, upset stomach, stomach pain, vomiting, gas, constipation, diarrhea, bloody vomit, bloody diarrhea or black, tarry stools, ringing in the ears, swelling of the hands, feet, ankles, or lower legs
Trade Name: Ansaid
Skin Effects: skin rash, itching

ibuprofen temporary relief of minor pain such as toothaches, muscular aches, minor arthritis pain, common cold, and menstrual cramps

Side Effects: facial swelling, wheezing, shock
Trade Names: Motrin, Advil
Skin Effects: skin reddening, rash, blisters

indomethacin for the treatment of moderate to severe pain associated with chronic rheumatoid arthritis, ankylosing spondylitis, osteoarthritis, bursitis, tendonitis, or gouty arthritis

Side Effects: nausea, vomiting, dyspepsia, indigestion, heartburn, epighastric pain, diarrhea, abdominal distress or pain, constipation, headache, dizziness, vertigo, somnolence, depression, fatigue, malaise, listlessness, tinnitus
Trade Name: Indocin
Skin Effects: pruritus, rash, urticaria, petechiae or ecchymosis

ketoprofen prescribed for the pain, tenderness, swelling, and stiffness caused by arthritis; useful in the treatment of other pain management, including the pain associated with muscle trauma, dental work, and childbirth; also, menstrual pain, postsurgical pain

Side Effects: headache, dizziness, nervousness, upset stomach, stomach pain or cramps, vomiting, constipation, diarrhea, gas, and less common side effects, including bloody vomit, bloody diarrhea or black, tarry stools, ringing in the ears, swelling of the feet, hands, ankles, or lower legs
Trade Names: Orudis, Actron
Skin Effects: skin rash and itching

ketorolac recommended for the treatment of moderately severe acute pain; provides pain relief at an opioid level; not indicated for minor pain or for those with chronic pain

Side Effects: peptic ulcers, GI bleeding, renal impairment, risk of bleeding, anaphylactic and anaphylactoid, liver failure, hypertension, nausea, dyspepsia, gastrointestional pain, diarrhea, constipation, flatulence, gastrointestional fullness, vomiting, stomatitis, headache, drowsiness, dizziness

Trade Name: Toradol
Skin Effects: pruritus, rash; less frequently, urticaria, sweating

meloxicam for the relief of pain associated with osteoarthritis and rheumatoid arthritis

Side Effects: abdominal pain, diarrhea, dyspepsia, flatulence, nausea, edema, flu-like symptoms, dizziness, headache, pharyngitis, upper respiratory tract infection
Trade Name: Mobic
Skin Effects: rash

nabumetone for treatment of acute and chronic pain associated with osteoarthritis and rheumatoid arthritis.

positive stool guaiac
test result that indicates the presence of blood in the stool

Side Effects: diarrhea, dyspepsia, abdominal pain, constipation, flatulence, nausea, **positive stool guaiac,** dry mouth, gastritis, stomatitis, vomiting, dizziness, headache, fatigue, insomnia, nervousness, somnolence, tinnitus, edema
Trade Name: Relafen
Skin Effects: sweating, pruritus, rash

naproxen for the treatment of pain associated with acute pain in situations such as severe dysmenorrhea, acute gout, rheumatoid arthritis, osteoarthritis, ankylosing spondylitis, juvenile arthritis, tendonitis, bursitis

Side Effects: heartburn, abdominal pain, nausea, constipation, diarrhea, dyspepsia, stomatitis, headache, dizziness, drowsiness, lightheadedness, vertigo, tinnitus, visuals disturbances, hearing disturbances, edema, palpitations, dyspnea, thirst
Trade Names: Anaprox, Naprosyn
Skin Effects: pruritus, skin eruptions, ecchymoses, sweating purpura

oxaprozin used to treat the symptoms associated with osteoarthritis and rheumatoid arthritis: pain, tenderness, stiffness, and swelling; can also be used for other types of pain

Side Effects: diarrhea, constipation, heartburn, upset stomach, vomiting, gas or bloating, stomach pain, drowsiness, difficulty sleeping, painful or frequent urination; more serious side effects include black and tarry stools, red blood in stools, bloody vomit, vomiting material that looks like coffee grounds, swelling of the hands, feet, ankles, or lower legs, unexplained weight gain, yellowing of the skin or eyes, fever, lack of energy, excessive tiredness, loss of appetite, difficulty breathing or swallowing, ringing in the ears

Trade Name: Daypro
Skin Effects: skin rash, itching, hives, pale skin

piroxicam used to relieve the pain, tenderness, stiffness, and swelling usually associated with arthritis

Side Effects: headache, dizziness, nervousness, upset stomach, stomach pain or cramps, vomiting, diarrhea, constipation, gas; bloody vomit, bloody diarrhea or black, tarry stools, ringing in the ears, swelling of the hands, feet, ankles, or lower legs
Trade Name: Feldene
Skin Effects: skin rash, itching

sulindac for the treatment of osteoarthritis, rheumatoid arthritis, ankylosing spondylitis, bursitis, **supraspinatus** tendonitis, acute gouty arthritis

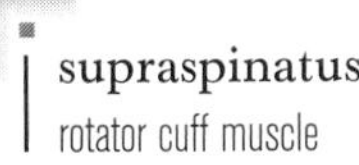

Side Effects: dyspepsia, nausea, vomiting, diarrhea, constipation, flatulence, anorexia, gastrointestinal cramps, dizziness, headache, nervousness, tinnitus, edema
Trade Name: Clinoril
Skin Effects: Stevens-Johnson syndrome, exfoliative dermatitis

tolmetin for the relief of pain associated with chronic diseases and the signs and symptoms of osteoarthritis and rheumatoid arthritis

Side Effects: nausea dyspepsia, gastrointestinal distress, abdominal pain, diarrhea, flatulence, vomiting, constipation, gastritis, peptic ulcer, headaches, asthenia, chest pain, hypertension, edema, dizziness, drowsiness, depression, changes in weight, tinnitus, visual disturbances, urinary tract infections
Trade Name: Tolectin
Skin Effects: skin irritation; less frequently but still possible: urticaria, purpura, erythema multiforme, toxic epidermal necrolysis

NON-NARCOTIC ANALGESICS

Non-narcotic analgesics are the most common pain relief medications used to treat pain from conditions such as osteoarthritis, partly because they cause few side effects. They are usually effective for people who have mild to moderate pain. Non-narcotic analgesics, such as acetaminophen, work by blocking pain centers in the brain. They also increase a patient's ability to withstand pain by increasing his or her pain threshold.

acetaminophen used for the relief of minor aches and pains, usually due to headache, muscular pain, backache, arthritis, common colds, toothaches, menstrual cramps

Side Effects: Allergic reactions can occur with Tylenol. If the following symptoms occur, they should be treated as an allergic reaction, and medical help is indicated: difficulty breathing, closing of the throat, swelling lips, tongue, and face, and hives. Liver damage can also occur with acetaminophen. This would be manifested by yellowing of the skin or eyes, nausea, abdominal pain or discomfort, unusual bleeding or bruising, or severe fatigue. Bleeding and bruising unrelated to liver damage can also occur.
Trade Name: Tylenol
Skin Effects: Hives and swelling are related to an allergic response and should be attended to by a medical professional.

butalbital compounds management of mild to moderate pain

Side Effects: drowsiness, hangover, insomnia, irritability, nausea, vomiting, angioedema, serum sickness, physical and psychological dependence
Trade Names: Esgic, Fioricet, Fiorinal, Phrenilin
Skin Effects: dermatitis, rash

capsaicin relief of mild to moderate pain associated with rheumatoid arthritis and osteoarthritis

Side Effects: cough
Trade Name: Zostrix
Skin Effects: burning

choline and magnesium salicylates relief of mild to moderate pain associated with rheumatoid arthritis and osteoarthritis

Side Effects: dyspepsia, epigastric distress, nausea, vomiting
Trade Names: CMT, Tricosal, Trilisate
Skin Effects: none

choline salicylates relief of mild to moderate pain associated with rheumatoid arthritis and osteoarthritis

Side Effects: dyspepsia, epigastric distress, nausea, vomiting
Trade Name: Arthropan
Skin Effects: none

magnesium salicylates relief of mild to moderate pain associated with rheumatoid arthritis and osteoarthritis

Side Effects: dyspepsia, epigastric distress, nausea, vomiting
Trade Names: Doan's Regular Strength, Magan
Skin Effects: none

salsalate relief of mild to moderate pain associated with rheumatoid arthritis and osteoarthritis

Side Effects: dyspepsia, epigastric distress, nausea, vomiting
Trade Name: Disaclid
Skin Effects: exfoliative dermatitis, Stevens-Johnson syndrome, toxic epidermal necrolysis

MUSCLE RELAXANTS

Muscle relaxants relax certain muscles in the body and relieve the stiffness, pain, and discomfort caused by strains, sprains, or other injury to muscles. However, these medicines do not take the place of rest, exercise or physical therapy, or other treatment that a doctor may recommend to treat the medical problem. Muscle relaxants act on the central nervous system to produce their effects. In the United States, these medicines are available only with a doctor's prescription.

baclofen treatment of severe **spasticity** resulting from multiple sclerosis

spasticity
pertaining to spasms or uncontrollable muscle movement

Side Effects: dizziness, drowsiness, fatigue, weakness, nausea
Trade Name: Lioresal
Skin Effects: sweating, rash, pruritus

carisoprodol relief of acute muscle spasms

Side Effects: dizziness, drowsiness, headache, nausea, vomiting, psychological dependence
Trade Name: Soma
Skin Effects: flushing and rashes

chlorzoxazone relief of acute muscle spasms

Side Effects: dizziness, drowsiness, diarrhea, nausea, vomiting
Trade Names: Paraflex, Parafon Forte DSC
Skin Effects: allergic dermatitis

cyclobenzaprine relief of acute muscle spasms

Side Effects: dizziness drowsiness, blurred vision, constipation, nausea
Trade Name: Flexeril
Skin Effects: none

dantrolene management of spastic activity associated with spinal cord injury, stroke, cerebal palsy, or multiple sclerosis

Side Effects: drowsiness, muscle weakness, headache, malaise, diarrhea
Trade Name: Dantrium
Skin Effects: pruritus, sweating, urticaria

diazepam anxiety management, relaxant, sedation, and chemical withdrawal

Side Effects: dizziness, drowsiness, lethargy, constipation, nausea, vomiting, phlebitis, physical dependence
Trade Name: Valium
Skin Effects: rashes

metaxalone relief of acute muscle spasms

Side Effects: drowsiness, dizziness, nausea, vomiting, dry mouth
Trade Name: Skelaxin
Skin Effects: none

methocarbamol relief of acute muscle spasms

Side Effects: dizziness, drowsiness, lightheadedness, loss of appetite resulting in weight loss, nausea, upset stomach
Trade Name: Robaxin
Skin Effects: flushing, pruritus, rash, urticaria

orphenadrine relief of acute muscle spasms

Side Effects: confusion, dizziness, drowsiness, blurred vision, constipation, dry mouth
Trade Name: Norflex
Skin Effects: none

Conclusion

Pain can be terrible to endure, but is the body's mechanism for signaling that something is wrong. Once the cause of pain is identified, pain management becomes necessary. Narcotic medications, non-narcotic medications, and nonsteroidal anti-inflammatory medications are the most widely used means of controlling pain from a pharmacologic perspective.

Along with these drugs come some side effects of which an aesthetician should be aware. Knowing the client's health history and the medications being used is vital. This knowledge helps assess the origin of a skin complaint, assists in evaluating a client's candidacy for certain treatments, and acts as a warning flag for referring the client to a physician.

REFERENCES

1. http://www.nlm.nih.gov
2. http://www.rxlist.com
3. http://www.drugs.com
4. Deglin, J. H., & Vallerand, A. H. (2007). *Davis's Drug Guide for Nurses.* Philadelphia, PA: F. A. Davis.
5. Michalun, N. (2001). *Milady's Skin Care and Cosmetic Ingredients Dictionary.* Clifton Park: Thomson Delmar Learning.
6. Spratto, G. R., & Woods, A. L. (2005). *2005 PDR Nurse's Drug Handbook.* Clifton Park: Thomson Delmar Learning.
7. http://www.fda.gov

Herbs, Vitamins, and Weight Control Drugs

CHAPTER 18

KEY TERMS

Adynamic Bone Disease
Cofactors
Enzymes
Holistic
Photophobia

LEARNING OBJECTIVES

After completing this chapter, you should be able to:

1. Define the different types of holistic treatments.
2. Define herbs, vitamins, and weight control medications.
3. Explain the side effects of herbs, vitamins, and weight control medications.
4. Explain the skin effects of herbs, vitamins, and weight control medications.

INTRODUCTION

With an aging society in the United States, it is important to consider as many lines of defense as possible to maintain good health and a good quality of life. For some, this encompasses searching for remedies that are more **holistic** in nature. As an adjunct component or a primary means of wellness, herbs and vitamins are used by millions of people to treat or prevent many conditions.

holistic
pertinent to the belief that entities are whole and cannot be limited to the function of their parts; use of natural remedies to cure disease

A major component of overall health is weight management. Maintaining a healthy weight is important for preventing a variety of conditions, including diabetes, heart disease, and bone deterioration. For individuals who do not see measurable results by dieting and exercising alone, their doctors can prescribe certain medications that will suppress their appetite or kick start their metabolism. In addition to medications that are prescribed by a physician, there are also remedies that can be purchased over the counter. These remedies have been left out of this text, as their benefits have not been evaluated or proven.

Similarly, most herbs and vitamins are available over the counter and are not evaluated by the FDA.

Finally, in the sections ahead you will notice the category *Trade Names* may contain only one or two trade names. There are many skin care products, almost too numerous to mention. Nevertheless, some examples are relevant; this listing is by no means an endorsement and should not be interpreted as such.

HERBS

Herbs have been used for a variety of means for thousands of years. Usages for herbs include fragrance, cooking, and, especially, wellness. In fact, the earliest medications were herbal. Today, most people use herbs to prevent many conditions, as well as treat disease without the complicated and often toxic complications associated with traditional prescription medications.

arnica herbal treatment for minor bone/ joint pain

Side Effects: hypersensitive reaction
Other Names: leopard's bane, mountain tobacco, mountain snuff, wolf's bane
Skin Effects: edematous dermatitis, eczema

black cohosh herbal treatment for menopause or premenstrual syndrome

Side Effects: headache, dizziness, upset stomach
Other Names: baneberry, black snakeroot, bugbane, rattle root, squawroot
Skin Effects: rash

chondroitin used to soften joint tissue for individuals with osteoarthritis or osteoporosis

Side Effects: heartburn, nausea, diarrhea
Other Name: chondroitin polysulfate
Skin Effects: allergic reaction, swelling, hair loss

dong quai herbal remedy for symptoms of menstrual cramping and menopause

Side Effects: may be carcinogenic
Other Names: Angelica sinensis, Dong Quai, Phytoestrogen
Skin Effects: photosensitivity

echinacea prevention and reduction of symptoms resulting from bacterial and viral infections

Side Effects: dizziness, fatigue, headache, nausea, vomiting, diarrhea
Other Names: American coneflower, black Sampson, black Susan, Kansas snakeroot, purple coneflower, Sampson root, scurvy root
Skin Effects: rash

feverfew taken orally to treat migraine headaches and used topically to relieve toothaches

Side Effects: headache, insomnia, nausea, diarrhea, vomiting
Other Names: Altamisa, Bachelor's Button, Chrysanthemum parethenium, Featherfew, Santa Maria, Wild chamomile
Skin Effects: contact dermatitis (orally only)

garlic used to prevent heart disease and colorectal and stomach cancers

Side Effects: dizziness, upset stomach, nausea, bad breath, bad body odor
Other Names: Alli sativa bulbus, Allium sativum
Skin Effects: contact dermatitis

ginger prevention and treatment of nausea and vomiting

Side Effects: heartburn

Other Names: Calicut, cochin, gengibre, ginger root, Jamaica ginger, kankyo, zenzero, zingiber
Skin Effects: dermatitis

ginkgo treatment of minor brain dysfunction including short term memory loss, as well as sexual dysfunction

Side Effects: dizziness, headache, seizure, palpitations
Other Names: Bai guo ye, fossil tree, folium, ginkgo biloba, Japanese silver apricot, kew tree, salisburia adiantifolia, yinsing
Skin Effects: rash, allergic reaction

ginseng improves mental and physical stamina

Side Effects: insomnia, agitation, nervousness, hypertension, tachycardia
Other Names: Asian ginseng, Chinese ginseng, hong shen, Japanese ginseng, Korean ginseng, red ginseng, renshen, white ginseng
Skin Effects: skin eruptions

glucosamine treatment of osteoarthritis often used in conjunction with chondroitin (see above; see Chapter 14 for more information)

Side Effects: nausea, heartburn, diarrhea, headache
Other Names: 2-amino-2-deoxyglucose sulfate, chitosamine
Skin Effects: skin eruptions

hawthorn herbal treatment for hypertension

Side Effects: dizziness, headache, vertigo, sedation
Other Names: aubepine, cum flore, hagedorn, maybush, whitehorn
Skin Effects: none

kava-kava herbal treatment for anxiety or insomnia

Side Effects: dizziness, drowsiness, visual disturbances, upset stomach, nausea, muscle weakness
Other Names: Ava pepper, intoxicating pepper, kao, kew, tonga, yagona
Skin Effects: allergic reactions, jaundice, pellagroid dermopathy

milk thistle herbal detoxifier/ liver cleanser

Side Effects: nausea, bloating, diarrhea
Other Names: Holy thistle, Lady's thistle, Mary Thistle, Silybin, Silymarin
Skin Effects: none

SAMe herbal treatment for a variety of conditions including depression, liver disease, osteoarthritis, and migraine headaches

Side Effects: agitation, dizziness, insomnia, vomiting, diarrhea, flatulence
Other Names: Ademetionine, S-adenosylmethionine
Skin Effects: none

saw palmetto used in combination with other herbs as a treatment for prostate cancer

Side Effects: dizziness, diarrhea, headache, constipation
Other Names: American Dwarf Palm, Cabbage Palm, Ju-Zhong, Palmier Nain, Sabal, Saw Palmetto Berry, Serenoa repens
Skin Effects: none

St. John's wort herbal treatment of depression and obsessive-compulsive disorder; also applied topically to treat blunt trauma wounds, burns, and inflammation of the skin

Side Effects: dizziness, sleep disturbances, constipation, dry mouth, nausea, vomiting
Other Names: Amber, Demon chaser, Goatweed, Rosin Rose, Tipton weed
Skin Effects: rash, pruritus, urticaria, photosensitivity

valerian herbal treatment of anxiety and insomia

Side Effects: drowsiness, headache
Other Names: Amantilla, All-Heal, Baldrian, Belgian Valerian, Common Valerian, Fragrant Valerian, Garden Heliotrope, Garden Valerian, Tagara, Valeriana officinalis, Valeriana rhizome, Valeriane
Skin Effects: none

VITAMINS

Vitamins are essential for normal metabolism, growth and development, and regulation of cell function. Vitamins work together with **enzymes**, **cofactors**, and other substances necessary for healthy life. There are two different types of vitamins: water-soluble and fat-soluble.

enzymes
agents that act as catalysts for many functions within the body; they act in coordination with chemicals, hormones, and other agents to allow for normal functioning

cofactors
agents that aid in the functioning of normal processes; often enzymes or hormones

Fat-Soluble Vitamins

Unlike water-soluble vitamins that need regular replacement in the body, fat-soluble vitamins are stored in the liver and fatty tissues and are eliminated much more slowly than water-soluble vitamins. Because fat-soluble vitamins are stored for long periods, they generally pose a greater risk for toxicity when consumed in excess than water-soluble vitamins.

While diseases caused by a lack of fat-soluble vitamins are rare in the United States, symptoms of mild deficiency can develop without adequate amounts of vitamins in the diet. Additionally, some health problems may decrease the absorption of fat and, in turn, decrease the absorption of vitamins A, D, E, and K.

alpha tocopherol (vitamin E) used topically to treat dry skin

Side Effects: (mostly due to overdose) headache, fatigue, cramps, diarrhea, nausea
Trade Names: Amino-Opti-E, Aquasol E, E-200, E-Complex 600, Liqui-E, Pheryl E, Vita Plus E
Skin Effects: rash

calcifediol vitamin D compound used for the treatment of metabolic bone disorders

Side Effects: hypercalcemia, headache, photophobia, decreased libido, bone pain, muscle pain
Trade Name: Calderol
Skin Effects: pruritus

calcitriol vitamin D compound used for the treatment of metabolic bone disorders, hypocalcemia, and chronic renal failure

Side Effects: hypercalcemia, headache, **photophobia**, decreased libido, bone pain, muscle pain
Trade Names: 1,25-dihydroxycholecalciferol, Calcijex, Rocaltrol, vitamin D3
Skin Effects: pruritus

photophobia
fear of light

adynamic bone disease
weakness or loss of bone strength

dihydrotachysterol vitamin D compound used in the treatment of hypocalcemia, as well as for the prevention and treatment of rickets

Side Effects: hypercalcemia, headache, photophobia, decreased libido, bone pain, muscle pain
Trade Names: DHT, Hytakerol
Skin Effects: pruritus

doxercalciferol vitamin D compound used to reduce elevated parathyroid hormone levels in dialysis patients

Side Effects: dizziness, sleep disturbances, dyspnea, bradycardia, hypercalcuria, **adynamic bone disease**

Trade Name: Hectorol
Skin Effects: pruritus

ergocalciferol (vitamin D2) vitamin D compound used for vitamin D deficiency

Side Effects: hypercalcemia, headache, photophobia, decreased libido, bone pain, muscle pain, palpitations, edema, allergic reactions, chills, fever
Trade Names: Calciferol, Deltalin, Drisdol
Skin Effects: pruritus

paricalcitol vitamin D compound used to treat and prevent hyperparathyroidism in patients with chronic renal failure

Side Effects: hypercalcemia, headache, photophobia, decreased libido, bone pain, muscle pain, palpitations, edema, allergic reactions, chills, fever
Trade Name: Zemplar
Skin Effects: pruritus

phytonadione (vitamin K) treatment and prevention of hypoprothrombinemia

Side Effects: bad taste
Trade Names: AquaMEPHYTON, Mephyton
Skin Effects: flushing, rash, urticaria, erythema, swelling

vitamin A helps form and maintain healthy teeth, skeletal and soft tissue, mucous membranes, and skin; also important to vision and reproduction

Side Effects: high cholesterol, liver damage, vision problems, fatigue, nausea (toxicity)
Trade Names: too numerous to list
Skin Effects: hair loss (toxicity)

Water-Soluble Vitamins

In contrast to the fat-soluble vitamins, the water-soluble vitamins are not easily stored by the body. They are often lost from foods during cooking or are eliminated from the body.

The water-soluble vitamins include vitamin C, which has been in the spotlight for many years and is best known for its ability to combat colds and for its function as an antioxidant. The B vitamins basically act as coenzymes and are involved in the metabolism of fat, protein, and carbohydrates.

The water-soluble vitamins are not normally stored in the body in any significant amounts. Therefore, they must be consumed in constant daily amounts to avoid depletion and interference with normal metabolic functioning.

ascorbic acid antioxidant and water-soluble vitamin necessary for many functions

Side Effects: upset stomach and diarrhea
Trade Names: Asorbicap, Cebid, Cecon, Cecore-500, Cemill, Cenolate, Cetane, Cevalin, Cevi-Bid, Flavorcee, Mega C/A Plus, Ortho/CS, Sunkist, Vitamin C
Skin Effects: none

cyanocobalamin (vitamin B12) treatment for B12 deficiency, which is important for metabolism and red blood cell formation

Side Effects: anemia, weakness, and loss of balance (deficiency)
Trade Names: Big Shot B-12, Cobex, Cobolin-M, Crystamine, Cyanoject, Cyomin, Nascobal, Primabalt, Rubesol-1000, Shovite, Vibal, Vitabee-12
Skin Effects: numbness or tingling in the extremities (deficiency)

folic acid water-soluble B vitamin vital to protein synthesis

Side Effects: inflammation of the tongue, mouth ulcers, peptic ulcer, diarrhea; may also lead to certain types of anemias, stomatitis, myelosuppression, and zinc depletion
Trade Names: too numerous to list
Skin Effects: graying of hair or alopecia (symptom of overdose)

hydroxocobalamin (vitamin B12) treatment for B12 deficiency, which is important for metabolism and red blood cell formation

Side Effects: anemia, weakness, and loss of balance (deficiency)
Trade Names: Alphamin, Hydrobexan, Hydro-Cobex, Hydro-Crysti-12, Hydroxy-Cobol, LA-12, Vibal LA
Skin Effects: numbness or tingling in the extremities (deficiency)

niacin (vitamin B3) important to the breakdown of carbohydrates, as well as promoting the health of the nervous system, skin, hair, eyes, mouth, and liver

Side Effects: indigestion, fatigue, canker sores, vomiting, depression (deficiency)

Trade Names: Edur-Acin, Nia-Bid, Niac, Niacels, Niacor, Niaspan, Nicobid, Nicolar, Nicotinex
Skin Effects: flushing (toxicity)

pantothenic acid (vitamin B5) important for skin, nerve, and lung function

Side Effects: none
Trade Names: Zest for Life, Now Foods, Country Life, Honey Combs, Twin Labs
Skin Effects: none

pyridoxine (vitamin B6) important for the breakdown of protein, fats, and carbohydrates

Side Effects: decreased sensation to touch, temperature, and vibration, poor coordination, fatigue
Trade Names: Beesix, Doxine, Nestrex, Pyri, Rodex, Vitabee 6
Skin Effects: numbness

riboflavin (vitamin B2) important to the production and health of many tissues within the body

Side Effects: discolored urine
Trade Names: Aqua-Flave, Beflavin, Beflavine, Bisulase, Dermadram, Fiboflavin, Flavaxin, Flavin, Flavin Bb, Flaxain, Hyflavin, Hyre, Lactobene, Lactoflavin, Lactoflavine, Lactoflavine, Zinvit-G, Ovoflavin, Ribipca, Ribocrisina, Riboderm, Riboflavin, Riboflavin 98%, Riboflavinequinone, Ribosyn, Ribotone, Ribovel, Russupteridine Yellow Iii, Vitaflavine
Negative Skin Effects: yellowing of the skin

thiamine (vitamin B1) essential for metabolizing carbohydrates, providing cardiovascular function, and producing energy

Side Effects: heart problems (deficiency)
Trade Name: Biamine
Skin Effects: none

Other Dietary Supplements

alpha lipo acid antiaging supplement that reverses signs of aging and improves overall body function

Side Effects: upset stomach, nausea, diarrhea, loose stools
Trade Names: Rosemary by Nature's Way, Syntrax-R, Natural Factors, Optimum Nutrition
Skin Effects: hypersensitive reaction

beta-carotene converted in the body to vitamin A, which is necessary for healthy eyes and skin

Side Effects: diarrhea, dizziness, joint pain
Trade Names: Lumitene, Max-Caro
Skin Effects: yellowing of the skin, unusual bleeding or bruising

biotin necessary for formation of fatty acids and glucose, which are used as fuels by the body; also important for the metabolism of amino acids and carbohydrates

Side Effects: none
Trade Names: Appearex, GCN, Meriben, Twin Labs
Skin Effects: none

choline necessary for the structure and function of all cells and important in the production of HDL (good) cholesterol

Side Effects: nausea, vomiting, bloating, diarrhea
Trade Name: Trilisate
Skin Effects: none

coenzyme Q-10 naturally occurring vitamin-like substance that possesses antioxidant qualities

Side Effects: headache, irritability, diarrhea, upset stomach (when taken orally)
Trade Name: Enovil
Skin Effects: erythema, pruritus, irritation

copper helps in the formation of red blood cells; also helps in keeping the blood vessels, nerves, immune system, and bones healthy

Side Effects: none; however, overdosing can lead to kidney problems
Trade Name: Cupri-Pak
Skin Effects: yellowing of the skin may indicate an overdose

iodine trace mineral essential to metabolism and production of thyroid hormones

Side Effects: mental retardation, hypothyroidism, goiter (deficiency)
Trade Name: Lugol's Solution
Skin Effects: yellowing of the skin (overdosing)

magnesium plays a role in the production and transport of energy; also important for the contraction and relaxation of muscles; involved in the synthesis of protein; assists in the functioning of certain enzymes in the body

Side Effects: muscle weakness, fatigue, irritability (deficiency)
Trade Names: Mag-Ox, Maox, Uro-Mag
Skin Effects: none

omega-3 fatty acid used to treat a variety of conditions including rheumatoid arthritis, high blood pressure, painful menstruation, and hay fever

Side Effects: bad taste, flatulence, diarrhea
Trade Names: Coromega, Long's Fish Oil, Max EPA, Omega-3, Salmon Oil, SuperEPA
Skin Effects: none

PABA (para-aminobenzoic acid) part of the vitamin B complex, it plays an import role in skin health and hormonal function; also used to treat certain skin conditions and is used as a UV block

Side Effects: fever
Trade Names: too numerous to list
Skin Effects: rash

potassium vital to electrical and cellular functions within the body

Side Effects: weakness, fatigue, cardiac arrhythmias, slow reflexes, and muscle weakness (deficiency), limited kidney function, abnormal breakdown of protein, and severe infection (overdose)
Trade Names: too numerous to list
Skin Effects: yellowing of the skin (overdose)

selenium vital to enzyme production and function

Side Effects: tooth loss, nausea, and fatigue
Trade Names: too numerous to list
Skin Effects: inflammation, hair loss, nail weakness

zinc plays important role in the proper functioning of the immune system in the body; required for the enzyme activities necessary for cell division, cell growth, and wound healing; plays a role in the acuity of the senses of smell and taste; also involved in the metabolism of carbohydrates

Side Effects: slow growth, poor appetite, impaired senses (deficiency)
Trade Names: too numerous to list
Skin Effects: skin lesions and infections, hair loss, impaired wound healing (deficiency)

Drugs Used on and for the Skin

CHAPTER 19

KEY TERMS

Antipruritic
Leukoderma
P. acnes
Psoriasiform
Tissue Necrosis

LEARNING OBJECTIVES

After completing this chapter, you should be able to:

1. Identify the skin problems that can be treated with a topical medication.
2. Define the drugs that are used to treat aesthetic skin concerns.

INTRODUCTION

As an aesthetician, you may work in a medi-spa or for a plastic surgeon. In either case, there is a host of prescription medications at your disposal. On the other hand, you may be one of the thousands of individuals who work in a day spa. Regardless of your chosen position, because antiaging prescription medications are commonly used today, it is important to know and understand these medications.

Aside from the prescription medications, there are also various vitamins and minerals that are not prescription, yet still have measurable effects on the skin. More so than most of the other medications that are contained within the pages of this book, these medications are the most commonly seen by the aesthetician.

These drugs, whether they are prescription or not, are delivered either systemically or topically. When used topically, the active ingredients work directly on the skin. A point that should be understood: *Most side effects of topical remedies are limited to the skin.* Some topical corticosteroids will have systemic side effects, but only rarely.

Finally, in the sections ahead you will notice the category *Trade Names* may contain only one or two trade names. There are many skin care products, almost too numerous to mention. Nevertheless, some examples are relevant; however, this listing is by no means an endorsement and should not be interpreted as such. Furthermore, most of the drugs in this chapter are topical medications. If there are medications that are taken orally or injected, these are noted as such.

Aging Skin

As an aesthetician, you will notice that the single most common skin complaint of the clients you see will be related to aging skin. In an increasingly age obsessed society, youthful appearances are a desired commodity. Especially when considering the aging of society, everyone wants to look younger, which is easier said than done.

There are products to help combat the aging process. Some of them are commonly available in OTC creams and remedies, while others require prescriptions. Some of the prescriptions discussed are topical, such as Retin-A, while others are injectable, such as Botox. Some of the medications in this section may also be taken orally; however, this chapter is dedicated to topical or injectable products. The information on oral vitamins and herbals is found in Chapter 18.

alpha-lipoic acid topical antioxidant that works to neutralize free radicals, improves skin texture, and may improve wrinkles

Side Effects: rare side effects
Trade Names: Reviva, NV Perricone MD
Skin Effects: rash, erythema, itching, hives

dimethylaminoethanol (DMAE) topical use to promote skin tightening

Side Effects: rare side effects
Trade Name: Skin Eternal Serum
Skin Effects: rash, itching, hives, erythema

glycolic acid topical alpha hydroxy acid used to improve the skin's appearance and texture; it may reduce fine lines and hyperpigmentation and improve other skin conditions such as acne

Side Effects: rare side effects
Trade Names: BioMedic LaRoche Posay, Aqua Glycolic, MD Formulations
Skin Effects: redness, burning, itching, hives

green tea topical antioxidant and anti-inflammatory that may have an affect on wrinkles

Side Effects: rare side effects
Trade Name: Pamela Hill Skin Care's Green Tea Moisturizer
Skin Effects: irritation, redness, peeling

hyaluronic acid topical used to add moisture to dry skin and smooth the stratum corneum

Side Effects: rare side effects
Trade Names: too numerous to mention
Skin Effects: redness, burning, itching, hives

idebenone topical synthetic version of the antioxidant Co Q10, which acts to neutralize free radicals

Side Effects: rare side effects
Trade Name: Prevage
Skin Effects: erythema, itching, burning, hives, irritation

kinetin topical natural growth factor proven to help prevent and repair signs of aging and sun damage

Side Effects: rare side effects
Trade Name: OSMOTICS' Kinetin Cellular Renewal Serum and Kinerase
Skin Effects: burning, itching, pain, hives, redness

lactic acid topical alpha hydroxy acid used to improve the skin's appearance and texture; it may reduce wrinkles, acne scarring, hyperpigmentation, as well as improve many other skin conditions

Side Effects: rare side effects
Trade Names: BioMedic AntiBac Acne Wash, Dermalogica Gentle Cream Exfoliant
Skin Effects: redness, burning, itching, pain, hives

peptides topical precursors to amino acids, used to treat aging skin

Side Effects: none noted
Trade Names: Bioque Serum, SuperMax Multi Peptide Skin Solution Serum
Skin Effects: redness, burning, itching, pain, hives

retinoids topical synthetic vitamin A developed for the treatment of various skin conditions, such as severe acne, psoriasis, sun spots, wrinkles

Side Effects: rare side effects
Trade Names: Retin-A, Renova
Skin Effects: red, edematous, blistered, or crusted skin, irritation, photosensitivity, redness, pruritus, peeling

sunscreen agents topical chemical sun blocks absorb UV energy before it affects the skin; examples are octyl methoxycinnamate or octyl salicylate or less used PABA

Side Effects: rare side effects
Trade Name: Banana Boat
Skin Effects: redness, irritation, itching, hives

sunscreen agents topical physical sun blocks reflect the UV energy before it affects the skin; examples are zinc oxide or titanium dioxide; reflect or scatter UV radiation before it reaches your skin

Side Effects: rare side effects
Trade Name: Total Block CoTZ
Skin Effects: redness, irritation, itching, hives

tocopherol (vitamin E) topical fat soluble vitamin that has antioxidant properties

Side Effects: rare side effects
Trade Name: Jan Marini
Skin Effects: skin hives, rash, or itchy or swollen skin

ubiquinone (Coenzyme Q10) topical agent naturally occurring vitamin-like substance that possesses antioxidant qualities

Side Effects: rare side effects
Trade Name: Vita-Co-Enzyme Pamela Hill Skin Care
Skin Effects: erythema, itching, hives, irritation

vitamin C topical topical skin care agent well known antioxidant that combats free radical damage

Side Effects: rare side effects
Trade Names: Vitamin C 10% and 20% Pamela Hill Skin Care
Skin Effects: burning, erythema, itching, redness, hives

Wrinkles

Wrinkled skin is a result of either sun damage or the sagging that comes with age. The physiologic result is a degradation of the dermis. Some of the treatments for this problem are found above in the aging category. Contained in this section are injectables that can treat deeper wrinkles.

botulinum toxin type A a purified protein produced by the *Clostridium botulinum* bacterium, which reduces the activity of the muscles that cause wrinkles to form over time; an injectable agent

Side Effects: headache, respiratory infection, flu-like symptoms, droopy eyelids, nausea, arrhythmia, and myocardial infarction; may inhibit neurotransmitter reception
Trade Names: Botox, MyoBloc
Skin Effects: skin rash, erythema, urticaria, **psoriasiform,** pruritus

psoriasiform
lesions that appear as psoriasis

tissue necrosis
dying skin or tissue

bovine collagen an injectable agent, produced from cowhide

Side Effects: lumps, bumps, **tissue necrosis**, failure to correct the lines
Trade Names: Zyplast, Zyderm I, Zyderm II
Skin Effects: bruising, temporary redness, swelling, tender skin

calcium hydroxylapatite an injectable agent

Side Effects: lumps, bumps, tissue necrosis, failure to correct the lines
Trade Name: Radiesse
Skin Effects: bruising, temporary redness, swelling, tender skin

human collagen an injectable agent

Side Effects: lumps, bumps, tissue necrosis, failure to correct the lines
Trade Names: CosmoDerm/CosmoPlast
Skin Effects: bruising, temporary redness, swelling, tender skin

hyaluronic acid naturally occurring substance that is used as a dermal filler to fill in wrinkles; an injectable agent

Side Effects: lumps, bumps, tissue necrosis, failure to correct the lines
Trade Names: Hylaform, Hylaform 2, Restylane, Captique
Skin Effects: bruising, temporary redness, swelling, tender skin

poly L-lactic acid an injectable agent

Side Effects: bumps, lumps, tissue necrosis
Trade Name: Sculptra
Skin Effects: bruising, temporary redness, swelling, tender skin

Pigmented Skin

Skin pigmentation disorders occur because the body produces either too much or too little melanin. Melanin production can increase or decrease beyond normal, creating a mottled appearance in the skin. This irregular pigmentation has origins in solar exposure, pregnancy, medications, and birth control. It can be frustrating, yet is a simple problem to solve. There are drugs both OTC and prescription that can treat pigmented disorders.

Hyperpigmentation occurs when melanocytes are overstimulated in a haphazard fashion. Such is the case in melasma gravidarum, commonly known as the "pregnancy mask." This results not just from pregnancy but from the use of birth control pills as well.

Hypopigmentation occurs when melanocytes no longer produce melanin, leaving areas of the skin without pigment, such as vitiligo and **leukoderma**.

leukoderma
without skin pigmentation

azelaic acid typically used for the topical treatment of acne; it also has skin lightening properties

Side Effects: rare side effects
Trade Name: Azelex
Skin Effects: burning, stinging, itching, dryness, peeling, redness

hydroquinone a skin lightening agent used topically

Side Effects: rare side effects
Trade Names: Alphaquin HP, Alustra, Eldopaque, Eldopaque Forte, Eldoquin, Eldoquin Forte, Esoterica, Esoterica Sensitive Skin, Glyquin, Glyquin-XM, Lustra, Melanex, Melanol, Melpaque HP,

Melquin HP, Melquin-3, Nuquin HP, Solaquin, Solaquin Forte, Viquin Forte

Skin Effects: redness, irritation, hives, itching, burning

kojic acid chemical skin lightening agent used topically

Side Effects: rare side effects
Trade Name: Reviva
Skin Effects: redness, irritation, hives, itching, burning

Actinic Keratosis

Actinic keratosis can be treated with topical agents to prevent its progression to skin cancers.

fluorouracil topically used for the treatment of actinic keratosis

Side Effects: rare side effects
Trade Name: Efudex
Skin Effects: burning, discoloration of skin, itching

imiquimod used for the topical treatment of actinic keratosis and genital warts

Side Effects: rare side effects
Trade Name: Aldara
Skin Effects: redness, irritation, hives, itching, burning

Acne

Acne is one of the most common conditions in the world. According to some estimates, 85–100 percent of the world's population experiences an outbreak of acne vulgaris at some point in their lives. Most often, this occurs during adolescence, when the body begins to produce more hormones. At this stage in life, acne is more common in men, but the tide turns in adulthood, when more women than men have adult acne.

Acne vulgaris will most often present in areas of the skin with the densest amount of sebaceous follicles. These locations include the face, the upper arms, the upper chest, and the upper back. Acne can be either inflammatory or noninflammatory in nature.[1] The noninflammatory expression is characterized by papules, open comedones (commonly called blackheads), or closed comedones (commonly called whiteheads). Inflammatory acne presents with papules, pustules, and nodules with obvious inflammation. Localized symptoms may include pain and tenderness.

[1]http://www.emedicine.com/derm/topic2

In medical terms, the onset of an acne lesion is thought to have several key factors. The first of these factors is called follicular epidermal hyperproliferation (excessive follicle growth). The exact cause of this is not yet known. Some suspect that the hormone androgen is responsible. Other hypotheses include changes in lipid composition or inflammation. Regardless of the cause, the end result is the clogging of the pore. The next factor that contributes to the formation of a lesion is excessive sebum production. This mechanism is controlled by several endocrine functions. Any one of these functions can be overstimulated due to fluctuating hormonal conditions, such as those that occur with menstruation, puberty, or pregnancy. With the excess sebum trapped in the sealed pore, conditions are ripe for bacteria to grow. The bacteria, **P. acnes,** promote inflammation, and the lesion forms.

P. acnes
Propionibacterium acnes, the bacteria that is thought to cause acne vulgaris

adapalene topical medication that operates by keeping skin pores clear

Side Effects: rare side effects
Trade Name: Differin
Skin Effects: burning sensation or stinging of skin, dryness and peeling of skin, itching of skin, redness of skin, worsening of acne

Table 19-1 Antibiotics used for Acne

Drug Name	Trade Name
Clindamycin	Cleocin-T, Cleocin, Clinda-Derm, Clindagel, Clindesse, ClindaMax, Clindets, CTS, Evoclin
Ciprofloxacin	Cipro, Cipro XR, Proquin XR
Demeclocycline	Declomycin
Doxycycline	Doryx, Monodox, Vibramycin, Vibra Tabs
Erythromycin	ERYC, ERY-Tab, Erythromycin Base Filmtab, PCE Dispertab
Levofloxacin	Levaquin
Minocycline	Arestin, Dynacin, Minocin, Myrac, Vectrin
Metronidazole	MetroGel, MetroCream, MetroLotion, Noritate
Tetracyclines	Achromycin, Actisite, Panmycin, Robitet, Sumycin, Tetracap, Tetracyn, Tetralan

azelaic acid typically used for the topical treatment of acne; it also has skin lightening properties

Side Effects: rare side effects
Trade Name: Azelex
Skin Effects: burning, stinging, itching, dryness, peeling, redness

benzoyl peroxide OTC topical remedy for acne

Side Effects: rare side effects
Trade Names: Benzac, Benzagel, BenzaShave, Brevoxyl, Clearasil, Clearplex, Desquam, Fostex, Neutrogena, Oxy, PanOxyl
Skin Effects: burning, stinging, itching, dryness, peeling, redness

isotretinoin oral retinoid used for the treatment of severe acne

Side Effects: red, itchy, dry, and inflamed eyes, dry mouth and nose, thinning of the hair, fatigue
Trade Name: Accutane
Skin Effects: dry skin, red, cracked, and sore lips

salicylic acid used topically to treat acne and other skin conditions

Side Effects: rare side effects
Trade Name: BioMedic La Roche Posay Conditioning Solution
Skin Effects: redness, irritation, itching, hives

sodium sulfacetamide topical agent with antibacterial properties used topically to hinder bacterial growth on the skin

Side Effects: rare side effects
Trade Names: Klaron, Novacet, Plexion, Sulfacet-R, Fostex, Acnederm
Skin Effects: dry skin, redness, warmth, swelling, itching, stinging, burning, or irritation of the treated area

tazarotene topical used to treat acne and psoriasis by making the skin less red and reducing the number and size of lesions of the skin

Side Effects: see skin effects
Trade Name: Tazorac
Skin Effects: dry skin, redness, warmth, swelling, itching, stinging, burning, or irritation of the treated area

Psoriasis and Eczema

Psoriasis is a noncontagious inflammatory skin and joint disorder that presents with edematous lesions on the skin. It is a chronic and recurrent condition with no known cause. Onset and flare-ups of the disease are thought to be genetic and environmental in nature, however. The intensity of the condition varies from person to person. It is estimated that approximately 3 percent of Americans suffer from this disease.

Eczema is a very common condition, and it affects all races and ages, including young infants. About 1–2 percent of adults have eczema, and as many as 20 percent of children are affected. It usually begins early in life, even before asthma or hay fever. Most affected individuals have their first episode before the age of 5 years. For some, the disease will improve with time. For others, however, eczema is a chronic or recurrent disorder. Although it can occur just once, it usually occurs on and off throughout life, or lasts the entire lifetime.

acitretin an oral retinoid used for the treatment of severe psoriasis

Side Effects: shakiness, dizziness, sweating, confusion, nervousness, sudden changes in behavior or mood, headache, numbness or tingling around the mouth, weakness, sudden hunger, clumsy or jerky movements, seizures, swollen or bleeding gums, excessive saliva, tongue pain, swelling, blistering, mouth swelling or blistering, stomach pain, diarrhea, increased appetite, difficulty falling or staying asleep, sinus infection, runny nose, dry nose, nosebleed, joint pain, tight muscles, excessive sweating, hair loss, changes in hair texture, dry eyes, loss of eyebrows or eyelashes, hot flashes, flushing
Trade Name: Soriatane
Skin Effects: pale skin, peeling, dry, itchy, scaling, cracked, blistered, sticky, or infected skin, brittle or weak fingernails and toenails, dandruff, sunburn, abnormal skin odor, weak nails, chapped or swollen lips

mycophenolate mofetil systemic immunosuppressant, often used to treat organ transplant recipients, but also used to control psoriasis

Side Effects: constipation, diarrhea, headache, heartburn, nausea, stomach pain, vomiting, weakness, dizziness, trouble sleeping
Trade Name: CellCept
Skin Effects: acne, skin rash

retinoids topical synthetic vitamin A developed for the treatment of various skin conditions, such as severe acne, psoriasis, sun spots, wrinkles

Side Effects: rare side effects
Trade Names: Retin-A, Renova
Skin Effects: red, edematous, blistered, or crusted skin, irritation, photosensitivity, redness, pruritus, peeling

Table 19-2 Topical Corticosteroids Used to Treat Skin Conditions

Drug Name	Trade Name
Alclometasone	Aclovate
Amcinonide	Cyclocort
Betamethasone	Alphatrex, Beben, Betatrex, Beta-Val, Dermabet, Diprolene, Diprosone, Luxiq, Maxivate, Occlucort, Teladar, Uticort, Valisone, Valnac
Clobetasol	Embeline E, Temovate
Clocortolone	Cloderm
Desonide	DesOwen, Tridesilon
Desoximetasone	Topicort
Dexamethasone	Aeroseb-Dex, Decadron, Decaspray
Diflorasone	Florone, Maxiflor, Psorcon
Fluocinolone	Bio-Syn, Derma-Smoothe/FS, Flucoet, Fluonid, FS Shampoo, Synalar, Synemol
Flucinonide	Fluocin, Licon, Lidex, Vanos
Flurandrenolide	Cordran
Fluticasone	Cutavate
Halcinonide	Halog
Halobetasol	Ultravate
Hydrocortisone	Acticort, Aeroseb-HC, Ala-Cort, Ala-Scalp, Alphaderm, Anusol HC, Bactine, CaldeCORT Anti-itch, Carmol HC, Cteacort, Cort-Dome, Cortenema, Corticaine, Cortifair, Cortifoam, Cortizone, Dermacort, Dermi-Cort, Dermtex HC, FoilleCort, Gynecort, HemrilHC, Hi-Cor, Hycort, Hydro-Tex, Hytone, LactiCare-HC, Lanacort 9-1-1, Lemoderm, Locoid, Nutracort, Orabase-HCA, Pandel, Penecort, Pharma-Cort, Prevex HC, Proctocort, Rhulicort, Synacort, Texacort, Westcort
Methylprednisolone	Medrol
Mometasone	Elocon
Prednicarbate	Dermatop
Triamcinolone	Aristocort, Delta-Tritex, Flutex, Kenalog, Kenonel

tazarotene topical treatment used to treat acne and psoriasis by making the skin less red and reducing the number and size of lesions of the skin

Side Effects: rare side effects
Trade Name: Tazorac
Skin Effects: burning or stinging of the skin, changes in color of treated skin, dryness, itching, peeling, or redness of the skin, pain or swelling, skin rash, burning or stinging after application

Dermatitis

Dermatitis is a delayed hypersensitive reaction to a material or substance with which the skin has come into contact. There are many causes for contact dermatitis. For every material in the world, there is someone who will have a hypersensitive reaction. In fact, there are entire volumes dedicated to the materials, environmental factors, and substances for which the hypersensitivity is caused. To this effect, a comprehensive discussion of this matter is beyond the scope of this text. However, a general overview of contact dermatitis is appropriate, as it is very common.

Contact dermatitis can be further subdivided into allergic contact dermatitis, irritant dermatitis, photo contact dermatitis, contact urticaria, and reactions to active pharmacologic agents. These subtypes are dependent upon the specific agent that causes the reaction.

Contact dermatitis is extremely common. It is consistently one of the top ten reasons for which people seek medical help. For example, as many as 30 million Americans will develop an allergic rash after coming in contact with antigens like poison ivy or poison sumac each year. Approximately 30 percent of all otherwise healthy children will experience a contact dermatitis episode over the course of their childhood. Among

Table 19-3 Subtypes of Contact Dermatitis

Subtype	Responsible Agent	Example
Allergic contact dermatitis	Allergens	Poison ivy or poison sumac
Irritant contact dermatitis	Irritants	Soaps or makeup
Photo contact dermatitis	Light sources	Sunlight
Contact urticaria	Allergens	Medications or plants
Reactions to active pharmacologic agents	Pharmacology agents	Benzocaine

workers' compensation claims for skin conditions, contact dermatitis accounts for 90 percent.

Typically, contact dermatitis is thought to infect Caucasians most often. Particularly fair skinned redheads are most susceptible. Also, women are twice as likely to experience contact dermatitis as men.

Most people will experience contact dermatitis in adulthood, but there are some generalizations that can be made. For instance, infants will experience contact dermatitis due to diaper rash, children will experience poison ivy in childhood more commonly (particularly boys), and adolescents will experience irritant contact dermatitis because of more common exposure to soaps and makeup.

flurandrenolide topical medication used to treat the itching, redness, dryness, crusting, scaling, inflammation, and discomfort of various skin conditions

Side Effects: rare side effects
Trade Name: Cordran
Skin Effects: drying or cracking of the skin, acne, itching, change in skin color

fluocinonide topical medication used to treat the itching, redness, dryness, crusting, scaling, inflammation, and discomfort of various skin conditions

Table 19-4 Common Sources for Contact Dermatitis
Poison ivy, oak, or sumac
Metals
Carbamates (rubber additive)
Thiurams
Imidazolinyl urea (in cosmetics)
Pet dander
Quaternium-15 (in cosmetics)
Fragrance additives
Alkalis
Acids
Wet cement

Side Effects: rare side effects
Trade Names: Fluonex, Lidex
Skin Effects: drying or cracking of the skin, acne, itching, burning, change in skin color

antipruritic
to cease itching

hydroxyzine **antipruritic** used orally to treat symptoms of dermatitis

Side Effects: dry mouth, nose, and throat, upset stomach, drowsiness, dizziness, chest congestion, headache
Trade Name: Atarax
Skin Effects: reddening of skin

pimecrolimus topical cream used to suppress the reactions associated with atopic dermatitis

Side Effects: rare side effects
Trade Name: Elidel
Skin Effects: burning, itching, redness; increased skin effects if this medication is combined with topical cortisones

Topical Drugs for Healing

There are a few topicals that are used on the skin to manage the healing process or prevent infection.

arnica used topically has an anti-inflammatory and analgesic effect on the skin

Side Effects: rare side effects
Trade Names: Arniflora Gel, Arnica Massage Oil, Arnicalm Arthritis, Arnicalm Trauma, ArnicAid
Skin Effects: redness, irritation, peeling, burning, stinging

Polysporin, Bacitracin, Neosporin used topically, has anti-infective properties

Side Effects: rare side effects
Trade Name: Triple Antibiotic Ointment
Skin Effects: hives, rash, redness, swelling

silver sulfadiazine cream primarily used to treat burns but also often used topically to treat wound injuries

Side Effects: rare changes in blood cell counts
Trade Name: Silvadene
Skin Effects: skin necrosis, erythema multiforme, changes in skin color, burning, rash

Conclusion

This chapter has focused on the medications that are used to treat the skin topically. Most of these medications do not have systemic side effects. The side effects are found at the site of the product application. If the skin becomes red or irritated with the use of a product, it is always sensible to discontinue the product while checking with the physician to ensure the reaction is unwanted.

REFERENCES

1. Van de Kerkhof, P. C. M. (2003). Psoriasis. In J. Bolognia, J. Jorizzo, & R. Rapini (Eds.), *Dermatology* (pp. 241–49). Philadelphia, PA: Mosby.
2. Kang, K., Poster, A., Nedorost, S., Stevens, S., & Cooper, K. (2003). Atopic Dermatitis. In J. Bolognia, J. Jorizzo, & R. Rapini (Eds.), *Dermatology* (pp. 199–213). Philadelphia, PA: Mosby.
3. Deglin, J. H., & Vallerand, A. H. (2007). *Davis's Drug Guide for Nurses.* Philadelphia, PA: F. A. Davis.
4. Mowad, C. M., & Marks, J. G., Jr. (2003). Allergic Contact Dermatitis. In J. Bolognia, J. Jorizzo, & R. Rapini (Eds.), *Dermatology* (pp. 227–39). Philadelphia, PA: Mosby.
5. http://www.nlm.nih.gov
6. http://www.rxlist.com
7. http://www.drugs.com
8. Michalun, N. (2001). *Milady's Skin Care and Cosmetic Ingredients Dictionary.* Clifton Park: Thomson Delmar Learning.
9. Spratto, G. R., & Woods, A. L. (2005). *2005 PDR Nurse's Drug Handbook.* Clifton Park: Thomson Delmar Learning.
10. http://www.fda.gov

Glossary

5-HT3 antagonists antienemic that is a selective serotonin inhibitor, which inhibits the binding of serotonin to 5-HT3 receptors

A

Acetylcholinesterase enzyme that inhibits the activity of acetylcholine

Acute coronary syndrome (ACS) general term used for any condition that causes chest pain resulting from limited blood flow to the heart

Acute hypoglycemia see hypoglycemia

Adrenocortical insufficiency suppression of one or more of the 50 plus hormones produced in the adrenal cortex

Adynamic bone disease weakness or loss of bone strength

Aldosterone adrenal cortex hormone responsible for metabolic regulation

Alopecia hair loss

Alpha-glucosidase Inhibitors group of medications used to treat diabetes by slowing the breakdown of sugars in the body

Alzheimer's Disease chronic, progressive neurological condition characterized by early onset of dementia

Anaphylactic reactions see anaphylaxis

Anaphylaxis serious hypersensitive allergic reaction characterized by respiratory distress, hypotension, edema, rash, and tachycardia. Immediate medical attention is necessary.

Angina chest pain resulting from lack of oxygen supplied to the heart

Ankylosing spondylitis stiffening of the vertebrae in the spine resulting in loss of movement

Anorexia condition characterized by weight loss stemming from a loss of appetite or refusal to eat

Antacid any agent that neutralizes stomach acid

Antianginals drug class that is used to prevent the onset of an angina attack

Antianxiety drugs any drug that prevents or limits the severity of the symptoms of an anxiety disorder

Antiasthmatics any drug that prevents or limits the severity of the symptoms of an asthma attack

Anticholinergics drug class that acts to limit spasms and cramping, particularly of the digestive and urinary tracts

Anticonvulsants any drug that prevents or limits the severity of spastic activity resulting from certain neurological conditions

Antidepressants any drug that prevents or limits the severity of the symptoms of depression

Antiemetics any drug that prevents or limits the severity of the symptoms of nausea and vomiting

Antigen any agent that provokes a hypersensitive reaction

Antihistamines any drug that blocks the action of histamine

Antipsychotics any drug that prevents or limits the severity of the symptoms of psychosis

Antispasmodics see anticonvulsants

Antiulcer drugs any drug that prevents or limits the severity of the symptoms of peptic ulcers

Aphthous stomatitis recurrent ulcers of the oral cavity

Apnea temporary ceasing of normal breathing function; can happen while sleeping

Arthralgia joint pain

Asthenia weakness or lack of strength

Asthma a chronic condition in which airway restriction results from a triggering event

Asymptomatic not presenting with any noticeable symptoms

Ataxia defective muscle coordination

Athlete's foot contagious fungal infection of the feet (also known as tinea pedis)

Atrial flutter cardiac arrhythmia characterized by a rapid activity of the atrial muscles

Atrioventricular conduction component of the cardiac electrical system

Atrophy loss of muscle tissue, most often from inactivity

Atypical unusual or dysfunctional

B

Barbiturates addictive central nervous system depressants

Benzodiazepines group of drugs with a sedative effect; predominantly used to treat anxiety and sleep disorders

Bipolar disorder mental condition characterized by periods of high activity and then severe depression

Blood lipids fat in the blood needed for normal functioning

Bronchodilators group of drugs that are used to reverse acute bronchial constriction

Bronchogenic cancers lung cancer that originates in the bronchus

C

Catechol-0-Methyltransferase inhibitors agents that break down levodopa, allowing greater availability in the central nervous system

Central nervous system stimulants any drug that increases central nervous system activity

Chloasma yellow or brown mispigmentation of the skin

Cholecystitis inflammation of the gall bladder

Cholelithiasis formation of gallstones

Cholinergic nerve endings that release acetylcholine

Chronic acid reflux disease recurrent condition characterized by stomach acids slipping into the esophagus resulting in a burning sensation in the chest; also known as GERD

Chronic metabolic acidosis condition characterized by the body having an abnormally low pH level

Clamminess sensation of the skin feeling cool to the touch

Claudication limping

Cofactors agents that aid in the functioning of normal processes; often enzymes or hormones

Congenital adrenogenital syndrome a condition characterized by overproduction of male hormones—occurring at birth. In females, this can result in the presence of male sex organs.

Conjunctivitis inflammation of the mucous membranes of the eyes and eyelids

Cyanosis bluish coloring of the skin resulting from reduced levels of hemoglobin in the blood

Cytomegalovirus retinitis type of herpes virus that can have potentially catastrophic effects on pregnancy

D

Depression condition characterized by low mood, loss of interest, loss of energy, weight changes, changes in appetite, changes in sleep patterns, fatigue, inability to concentrate, feelings of low self-worth, and possibly thoughts of suicide

Desquamation normal sloughing of the epidermis

Diastolic period in the cycle of the heartbeat in which the heart is at rest

Diplopia seeing double

Dopamine neurotransmitter whose performance is involved in many mental disorders

Dopamine agonists any agent that increases dopamine activity

Dowager hump a bump that forms along the spine occurring due to slow bone loss over time. This most commonly occurs in the elderly.

Dysmorphic abnormally formed

Dyspepsia symptomatic condition characterized by abnormal or painful digestion

Dysphoria feelings of depression, discomfort, or unhappiness with no known cause

Dysthymia chronic and mild depression often occurring from secondary antagonists (i.e., side effect from medication)

E

Ecchymoses bruising

Eczematoid dermatitis itchiness and redness of the skin resulting from eczema

Electrolytes any solution that conducts electricity in the body, most commonly salts, potassium, and chlorine

Endometriosis disease of the endometrium resulting in loss of tissue

Endometrium the mucous membrane lining the interior walls of the uterus

Enzymes agents that act as catalysts for many functions within the body; they act in coordination with chemicals, hormones, and other agents to allow for normal functioning

Epidermal necrolysis tissue death on the epidermis

Epilepsy neurologic condition characterized by sudden seizures

Erosive esophagitis condition characterized by the eroding of the esophagus; most commonly caused by chronic acid reflux disease

Erythema multiforme condition characterized by macular eruptions in a patchy formation on the extremities

Erythema nodosum characterized by tender, red bumps, usually found on the shins. Quite often, erythema nodosum is not a separate disease, but, rather, a sign of some other disease, or of a sensitivity to a drug.

Essential hypertension high blood pressure without a known cause

Etiology the study of the cause of a disease

Euphoria temporary state of excitement and happiness

Exanthema any inflamed skin eruptions

Extrapyramidal existing outside of the pyramidal tracts of the central nervous system

F

Flatulence excessive gas

G

Galactorrhea excessive milk flow beyond the completion of nursing

Generalized Anxiety Disorder (GAD) condition characterized by unspecific or unwarranted anxiety

Gingival hyperplasia overgrowth of the gums

Gingival hypoplasia underdevelopment of the gum tissue

Glucose vital sugar required for normal metabolism

Granulocytopenia abnormally low levels of granulocytes in the blood

Gynecomastia development of abnormally large breasts in men, which may secrete milk

H

Hallucinations symptom in which an individual sees or hears things that are not actually there

Hand and foot syndrome condition characterized by painful lesions on the hands and feet

Hantavirus virus that is transmitted to humans through mice feces with potentially fatal consequences

Health History Sheet document used by medical professionals to gather information on past and present health conditions, as well as likelihood for future conditions. This includes allergies, medical conditions, and prescription information.

Hemolytic anemia low iron levels resulting from the destruction of red blood cells

Hemoptysis coughing up blood

Hirsutism condition characterized by excessive hair growth in unusual places

Histamine protein in the body that stimulates hypersensitive reactions

Hodgkin's disease malignant tumor of the lymph system

Holistic pertinent to the belief that entities are whole and cannot be limited to the function of their parts; use of natural remedies to cure disease

Hydantoin anticonvulsants drugs that are most commonly used in the treatment of seizures associated with epilepsy

Hyperacidity condition in which the body produces too much acid

Hypercalcemia high blood calcium

Hyperchloremic acidosis condition characterized by increased chlorine levels resulting in higher acidity levels overall

Hypercholesterolemia condition characterized by abnormally high levels of cholesterol in the body

Hyperglycemia increased blood sugar levels often leading to diabetic coma if unresolved

Hyperkalemia abnormally high levels of potassium in the blood

Hyperlipidemia abnormally high levels of fat in the blood

Hyperpigmentation overproduction and overdeposits of melanin

Hyperplasia excessive proliferation of normal cells in tissue

Hypertension high blood pressure

Hypertrichosis excessive overgrowth of hair

Hyperuricemia abnormally high levels of uric acid in the blood

Hypocalcemia abnormally low levels of calcium in the blood

Hypoglycemia abnormally low levels of glucose in the blood

Hypogonadism condition characterized by underdevelopment of the gonads and secondary sexual characteristics

Hypokalemia abnormally low levels of potassium in the blood

Hypomagnesemia abnormally low levels of magnesium in the blood accompanied by muscle irritability

Hypopigmentation lack of production of melanin from melanocytes

Hypotension low blood pressure

Hypovolemia abnormally low water levels in the body

I

Immunocompromised referring to limited or reduced functioning of the immune system

Immunologic response process by which the body reacts to a perceived bacterial or viral threat and acts to eliminate it or neutralize it

Incretin mimetic agent a drug that is intended to trick the body into producing insulin as a means of treating diabetes

Insulin essential hormone needed for the normal metabolic breakdown of glucose in the body

Insulin dependent diabetes mellitus (IDDM) type of diabetes in which the body cannot produce insulin, or insulin is ineffective, resulting in the need for external supplies of insulin to be introduced (also known as Type 1 diabetes).

Irritable bowel syndrome condition characterized by disturbances of normal bowel function of unknown etiology

Ischemia temporary restriction in normal blood flow

J

Jaundice yellowing of the skin most often caused by improper liver functioning

K

Kaposi's sarcoma condition characterized by multiple areas of cell proliferation that eventually become cancerous

Ketoacidosis acidosis caused by abnormally high levels of ketone bodies, a compound that is a by-product of fat metabolism

L

Lethargy feelings of excessive sluggishness

Leukemia a malignant cancer of the blood producing tissues

Leukopenia unusual decrease in white blood cells

Leukotriene antagonist agent that acts as an inhibitor of leukotrienes, a chemical mediator of inflammation

Libido sexual desire

Lipodystrophy loss of fatty tissue due to defective fat metabolism

M

Maculopapular eruptions of both macules and papules

Major depression most severe type of depression characterized by severe and frequent instances of low mood, loss of interest, loss of energy, weight changes, changes in appetite, changes in sleep patterns, fatigue, inability to concentrate, feelings of low self-worth, and possibly thoughts of suicide

Meglitinides type of type 2 diabetes treatment that increases insulin production in the pancreas

Melasma general name for discoloration of the skin

Mental illness umbrella term for any condition that results in a measurable dysfunction of mental or psychotic functioning

Metabolic alkalosis increased alkalines in the body resulting from decreased acids

Metabolism the body's means of processing food into energy

Metastatic movement of cancer cells from one part of the body to another

Monoamine oxidase inhibitors (MAOIs) drug treatment for depression. The exact mode of their action is not quite understood.

Morbilliform resembling measles

Mottling skin condition characterized by discoloration of the skin

Mucocutaneous toxicity poisoning of the skin and mucous membranes

Mucositis inflammation of the mucous membranes

Multiple myeloma malignant neoplastic condition characterized by tumor cells infiltrating the bone and bone marrow

Myalgia muscle pain

Mycosis fungoides a rare t-cell skin cancer

Myelogenous originating in the bone marrow

Myocardial ischemia temporary restriction in normal blood flow to the heart and cardiac muscles

N

Narcotic a drug that is both physically and psychologically addictive, but has medicinal benefits

Nasopharyngitis inflammation of nasopharynx

Nephropathy kidney disease

Nephrotoxicity kidney toxicity

Neuroblastoma a certain type of malignant tumor originating in neuroblast cells of the brain

Neurogenic bladder improper bladder functioning resulting in overactivity or underactivity of normal urinary function

Neuroleptic drugs any medication that has side effects that resemble symptoms of neurologic diseases

Neuropathy disease of the brain or brain function

Neutropenia abnormally low levels of neutrophil cells in the body

Nocturia excessive and frequent urination at night

Non-Hodgkin's lymphoma a certain type of malignant cancer originating in the lymphatic system

Non-insulin dependent diabetes mellitus type of diabetes in which the body cannot utilize insulin, resulting in the need for monitoring or diet and exercise in addition to medication (also known as type 2 diabetes)

Norepinephrine hormone produced in the adrenal medulla that acts as a vasoconstrictor

Normal sinus rhythm an electrical impulse that regulates the normal heartbeat—usually at a pace of 60–100 beats per minute

Nystagmus involuntary and constant movement of the eyeball

O

Obsessive-compulsive disorder (OCD) anxiety disorder characterized by perpetual and excessive thoughts and activities that interfere with the normal functioning of the affected individual

Oligohydrosis condition characterized by excessive low water levels in the body

Oligospermia low sperm count

Oliguria lessening in the amount of urine

Onychomycosis parasitic infection of the nails

Opportunistic mycoses any fungus that uses discontinuations in the skin or abnormal immunity to infect the body

Osteoarthritis joint condition characterized by inflammation of weight-bearing joints

Overactive bladder condition characterized by abnormally high levels of bladder activity resulting in frequent need to urinate

Over-the-counter (OTC) a medication that is available for consumption without a physician's prescription

P

Paget's Disease condition affecting the elderly characterized by inflammation of the bones

Palmar-plantar erythrodysesthesia condition characterized by redness and pain on the palms and soles of the feet

Pancreatitis condition characterized by inflammation of the pancreas

Parenteral any drug delivery route other than oral

Paresthesia sensation of numbness and prickling; often called "pins and needles"

Parkinson's Disease nervous system condition characterized by progressive tremors, muscular weakness, and rigidity

Pathogenic fungi any fungus that results in disease

Peptic ulcer a wearing down of normal tissue of the stomach and esophagus, resulting in frequent stomach pain, especially after eating

Perioral around the mouth

Peripheral edema occurring away from; in this case swelling away from the trunk of the body; in the legs

Phenothiazines type of drug used to treat schizophrenic disorders

Phlebitis inflammation of a vein

Phobias anxiety condition characterized by unwarranted fear such that it interferes with the normal functioning of the affected individual

Photophobia fear of light

Photosensitivity condition characterized by increased sensitivity to light and the effects of light, particularly sunlight, on the skin

Physical dependence chemical dependence in which the body thinks it needs a substance in order to function

Pleural effusion fluid leakage in the thoracic cavity

Pneumonitis inflammation of the lungs

Porphyria cutanea tarda genetic condition characterized by a disruption in normal polyphyrin metabolism

Positive stool guaiac test result that indicates the presence of blood in the stool

Post-traumatic stress disorder anxiety condition that is the result of stress brought on by a traumatic event

Precocious puberty early onset of puberty

Prehypertension state of being on the verge of clinic hypertensive

Prescription a doctor's order for a medication in order to remedy an illness or the symptoms of an illness

Priapism a prolonged erection with the absence of sexual desire

Primary hypercholesterolemia the first in a series of events in which the affected individual presents with high cholesterol

Primary hypertension the first in a series of events in which the affected individual presents with high blood pressure

Prosthetic replacement of a missing part with a man-made substitute

Proteinuria high levels of protein in the urine

Proton pump inhibitors any antiulcer agent that restricts the acid production in the stomach

Pruritus itching

Psychological dependence type of chemical dependence characterized by the affected individuals thinking they need a substance for normal functioning

Psychosis most extreme cases of mental disturbance in which the affected individual has partially or totally lost touch with reality, either permanently or temporarily

R

Rebound hypoglycemia phenomenon associated with decreased glucose levels following the external introduction of insulin into the body for individuals with diabetes

Renal failure inability of the kidneys to function normally

Rigors hardness or stiffness of the muscles

S

Schizophrenia personality disorder characterized by a disassociation from social experience and limited social range

Seborrhea condition characterized by excessive sebaceous secretion

Select serotonin reuptake inhibitors (SSRIs) type of antidepressant that allows for more productive use of the neurotransmitter serotonin

Serotonin neurotransmitter that is thought to be a major contributor to many mental illnesses including depression, anxiety disorders, and personality disorders

Social phobias fear of public places or interacting with other people, which results in the need to avoid that which interferes with normal functioning

Spasticity pertaining to spasms or uncontrollable muscle movement

Specific phobias fear of a certain thing that results in the need to avoid that which interferes with normal functioning

Stevens-Johnson Syndrome see erythema multiforme

Subcutaneous mycoses a fungus that occurs under the skin

Sublingual under the tongue

Superficial mycoses usually result from the introduction of vegetative matter to an open wound; infection is limited to the dermis

Supraspinatus rotator cuff muscle

Syncope a momentary loss of blood flow to the brain, resulting in unconsciousness; fainting

Systemic antifungals antifungal medications that are ingested and distributed via the bloodstream

Systemic mycoses a fungus that affects the internal organs

Systolic period in the cycle of the heartbeat in which the heart is contracting

T

Tachycardia abnormally rapid heartbeat; usually over 100 beats per minute

Thrombocytopenia abnormal decrease in blood platelet levels

Tic a spastic muscle contraction, usually involving the face

Tinea capitis fungal infection of the scalp

Tinea corporis fungal infection of the skin on the body (also known as ringworm)

Tinea cruris fungal infection of the area surrounding the genitalia (also known as jock itch)

Tinnitus ringing in the ears

Topical antifungals any antifungal medication that is applied on top of the skin

Toxic epidermal necrolysis see epidermal necrolysis

Tricyclics (TCAs) the most commonly prescribed type of antidepressants used to treat the milder cases of depression or anxiety

Trigeminal neuralgia nerve pain along the nerves of the face

U

Unicellular pertaining to only one cell

Urticaria hives

V

Valproates anticonvulsants drugs that are meant to limit the frequency and severity of spastic activity

Vasodilation an increase in the flow capacity of veins

Vasopressin hormone that increases blood pressure

Ventricular arrhythmias irregular heartbeat that has its origin in the ventricular chambers of the heart

Ventricular tachycardia irregularly rapid heartbeat that is caused by the pumping of the ventricular chambers of the heart

Vertigo sensation of moving through space or of having objects float independently around. Often synonymous with dizziness

Virilism the presence of male patterned hair growth on women

Vitreous hemorrhage bleeding in the eye

Index

A

B

D

H

I

M

R

S

Z